MEMORY WISE

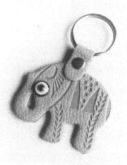

T0323111

DR ANNE UNKENSTEIN, PhD, is a clinical neuropsychologist who has focused on working with people who experience change in their memory. For over 25 years, Anne worked in a memory clinic at a large public hospital in Melbourne. She has also worked in public and private inpatient and community-based psychiatric health services, and consults in private practice. Her clinical work involves identifying the nature and extent of people's memory issues, assisting with the diagnosis of memory illnesses such as dementia, and providing supportive strategies for people with memory difficulties and their families. She holds an honorary position within the Department of Psychiatry at the University of Melbourne, and has been involved in the education of graduate neuropsychologists and psychiatrists. Anne's recent research, based at the Royal Women's Hospital in Melbourne, focused on women's experience of memory during the menopause transition, and enhancing women's memory self-confidence through the provision of group memory-strategies programs. Anne has presented her research at Australian and international scientific conferences and published her work in international journals and books. She has made educating the community about memory a priority throughout her career, contributing written information about memory and dementia to newsletters, websites and 'help sheets', and giving regular presentations through Dementia Australia, Council on the Ageing, community organisations, television and talk-back radio.

How memory works
and what to do
when it doesn't

MEMORY
WISE

DR ANNE UNKENSTEIN

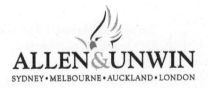

ALLEN&UNWIN
SYDNEY•MELBOURNE•AUCKLAND•LONDON

First published in 2019

Copyright © Anne Unkenstein 2019

All rights reserved. No part of this book may be reproduced or transmitted in any form or by any means, electronic or mechanical, including photocopying, recording or by any information storage and retrieval system, without prior permission in writing from the publisher. The Australian *Copyright Act 1968* (the Act) allows a maximum of one chapter or 10 per cent of this book, whichever is the greater, to be photocopied by any educational institution for its educational purposes provided that the educational institution (or body that administers it) has given a remuneration notice to the Copyright Agency (Australia) under the Act.

Allen & Unwin
83 Alexander Street
Crows Nest NSW 2065
Australia
Phone: (61 2) 8425 0100
Email: info@allenandunwin.com
Web: www.allenandunwin.com

A catalogue record for this book is available from the National Library of Australia

ISBN 978 1 76029 638 4

Set in 12.1/16.2 pt Minion Pro by Bookhouse, Sydney
Printed and bound in Australia by Griffin Press, part of Ovato

10 9 8 7 6 5 4 3 2

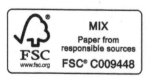

The paper in this book is FSC® certified. FSC® promotes environmentally responsible, socially beneficial and economically viable management of the world's forests.

In memory of Delys Sargeant AM
18 November 1927 – 19 September 2017

Contents

Introduction

At a particularly busy time in my life, when I was in my early thirties, I was working from home in the company of my four-year-old daughter. I had one day left to put the finishing touches on a project, and I was trying to squeeze in some writing in the morning. I put the kettle on to make a cup of tea, settled my daughter in front of her favourite television show, and went to my desk. After a little while I started to smell smoke. Suddenly I remembered the kettle! Oh no! I rushed into the kitchen and found the kettle boiled dry and burning on the gas stovetop. Later, after my shock had subsided, I bought a new electric kettle that turned itself off after it had boiled the water!

We all have memory lapses, at any age. When I boiled the kettle dry I was upset to think that I could have started a house fire, but I wasn't concerned about my memory. I knew that I had forgotten about the kettle because I was distracted by my inner 'to do' list and work deadline stress, and by my daughter in the adjacent room. But if I was older, say 65, then maybe I might start to worry about my memory, especially if I had forgotten a few other things that week too. Or if I was living on my own at 75, and I told my adult daughter about what happened, she might become concerned about me, and wonder if I had early signs of dementia.

It is common to feel worried about memory, but how do you know if memory difficulties are normal, or the beginnings of dementia? Does your ability to remember change as you get older? Can dementia be prevented? Where do you go if you have concerns about memory? What can we do to get the most out of our memory abilities?

This book was written to answer these sorts of questions. In fact, two previous versions of this book (originally named *Remembering Well*) were written about twenty years ago by a much younger me, together with my friend and mentor Delys Sargeant. Without Delys, this book would not exist. Sadly, in 2017 Delys died, aged 89. Delys was a health promotion activist, dedicated to educating health professionals and the community, and providing advice to government and health agencies on ageing, women's health and public health.

When Delys was in her late sixties, she became concerned about her memory and consulted me to have her memory assessed. The results were reassuring, and Delys decided to use her experience to help others who had similar concerns. Delys and I went on to provide regular community seminars on memory and ageing. After attendees asked what books they could read on the topic, we decided to write our own, and the first edition of *Remembering Well* was published in 1998, followed by a second edition in 2001. *Remembering Well* won the *Australasian Journal on Ageing*'s book award in 1999, was published in Spanish in Mexico, and an audio version was produced.

Delys and I were delighted to know that our book had been so warmly received, and had given emotional and practical help to readers who were concerned about their memory, or the memory abilities of a family member or friend. The main response from people who read the book was typically: 'I feel so much better now. I recognise that I do have strategies I can draw on as needed.' We heard with delight of one woman who had started to give the book to all her friends when they turned 50!

I have now worked as a clinical neuropsychologist, focusing on memory loss, for 30 years. For most of my career I have worked in memory clinics, seeing people who have memory issues that range from mild to severe, and working together with family members to foster personalised support. I have conducted research into memory, particularly for women during menopause. I have run memory courses for groups of people, helping them to identify aspects of life that make memory fluctuate, and taught practical techniques for managing memory change. My work has crossed over into my personal life. Now in my fifties, I am experiencing normal glitches in my own memory, and members of my family have experienced more significant memory loss, related to memory illnesses. Through both my work and my personal life, I have learned that we can wisen up to memory and manage it more efficiently.

Memory-wise focuses primarily on the everyday remembering that is such an important part of our lives. School children have to remember names, places, timetables, formulae, and words of songs. In the world of work, we rely on our memory for specific information and names of contacts. At leisure, we may need to remember cards at bridge, recall words for crossword puzzles, or names of old films or pieces of music. We remember technical procedures like how to drive a car, fix a fuse or set up a spreadsheet. At home, we need to know addresses, birthday dates and where we left the car keys. The list goes on. Every hour of the day we're calling on memory. Our capacity to respond to these demands depends on our state of mind at the time, on our health and, to some extent, on our age. We live in a busy, multi-tasking society, we work long hours, and we work to an older age. We deal with stress, overload, mental and physical health issues, and we don't get enough sleep. It's no wonder we notice changes in our memory!

Whenever I talk about memory in the community, large numbers of people come to listen and to discuss their concerns. This need to know about memory is increasing as the proportion of older people in our society continues to rise rapidly. Not only do we have more people around us who experience normal age-related memory change, we also have more people among us who have significant memory loss related to memory illnesses, such as dementia. As more people have first-hand experiences with relatives and friends who have dementia, and as dementia becomes an increasingly high-profile issue in the media, it is more likely that those who experience everyday memory lapses will become concerned that they have dementia.

The broad aim of this book is to provide practical information and advice for anyone who is concerned about their own memory, or the memory abilities of someone close to them. The book uses real-life stories (names and identifying details changed, except for mine) for illustration and is based on the original *Remembering Well*, with updated versions of all previous chapters and two new chapters.

Chapter 1 provides a framework for understanding how memory works. Chapter 2 describes changes that can occur in memory as we get older, along with continued strengths in some aspects of remembering. Health, attitude and lifestyle factors that can lead to fluctuations in memory are described in Chapter 3, together with practical tips to minimise the effect of these aspects of our lives on our memory. Chapter 4 focuses on memory during meno-pause, including recent research on women's memory performance at midlife. Researchers are continuing to update our knowledge on potential ways that we can reduce our risk of developing dementia, and Chapter 5 outlines practical suggestions for maintaining brain health based on current research.

We can all become more skilled in managing memory and more confident that we will remember. Chapter 6 describes prac-tical everyday strategies to help get the most out of our memory. Working and Learning (Chapter 7) is for those who want to enhance their memory at work, or learn new tricks, as part of a new job, voluntary work or new interests.

Fortunately, the majority of older people do not develop dementia, but as a community we need to be aware of more significant memory loss that occurs with memory illnesses such as dementia. Chapter 8 discusses the emotional reactions involved in a diagnosis of dementia and provides practical strategies for the person who has the illness in its early stages. Chapter 9 is written for friends and relatives who want to understand this early stage and how they might help. The book concludes with the proposal that we develop a memory-wise community (Chapter 10), in which we acknowledge and support memory change.

All of the chapters are designed to stand on their own, as well as offer cumulative understanding, so some repetition is inevitable, but hopefully this in itself will be a useful memory-wise strategy! Places you might go to for further advice about memory issues are suggested—but remember that health systems are not all the same, and memory clinics, or the role of doctor and neuropsychologist, for example, will vary according to where you live.

Memory change is a reality over the whole of our lives. This book explains how memory works—and what to do when it doesn't. Use it as a starting point to understand and nurture your own memory, and to help us all to live in a memory-wise community.

CHAPTER 1

How memory works

It is tempting to make all-or-none statements about memory as if it were a single concept. You might say, 'My memory is letting me down', for example—but is it a problem with remembering what you did yesterday, or what you did when you were a child? If a person is said to have a 'fantastic memory', is it for remembering names, or for recalling faces? Is the same process at work when we recall facts and figures, as when we register a familiar aroma—the salty sea air, gum trees, a roast in the oven—and it triggers a burst of feelings and memories we thought we had forgotten? What about community memory, represented in things like commemorative stamps, statues and symbols, in oral history, and in language itself?

Memory is mediated by culture: in some societies much more value is assigned to, say, musical memory skills, visualisation or the ability to remember complex dance movements than in others. Memory is individual: some of us remember the feelings and sense of events rather than the specific details; others have strong recall for facts and figures and are great to have on your team in a trivia quiz! Memory teamwork can work well, with an excellent memory for names complementing a strength in recognition of people's faces.

I'm not good at remembering jokes and trivia, but I can usually rely on my visual memory. This comes in handy when my children are rushing out the door saying, 'Has anyone seen my shoes?' I can often drum up a distinct memory of the shoes under the couch, where they were left the night before!

Maria, 44

My sister has a fantastic memory for facts and details. She is a lawyer and needs to be able to recall this type of information for her work. I'm different. I remember the feeling of things. I will go to a party, and forget what was said in the speeches or the name of the venue where the party was held, but I will remember the emotions that I felt whilst I was there and that it was a joyous occasion. I have always been like this.

Lucy, 62

Memory is, in fact, a very complex phenomenon: a whole book could be written outlining the current theories and debate about how memory works and its neurophysiological basis. The words that are used to describe various memory processes can be confusing, with terms like 'short-term memory' and 'long-term memory' meaning different things for different people. Without getting too technical, let's run though a simple model of memory to clarify memory terminology and to help understand which parts of the 'works' could need special care and attention.

The starting point is to think of memory as a storage system. Storage facilities are all around us: the refrigerator, the pantry, wardrobes, computers, smartphones, libraries, even department stores. Of course, some systems are more streamlined than others—locating a particular item in a library is usually much easier than finding the thing you want in your junk room!—but the procedures for using them are the same. Think of your good old filing cabinet: you put your selected work-related documents, family budgeting information or recipes into labelled folders, you store them in the cabinet, and you get them out when you want them. In other words, you *acquire* information, you *store* information and you *recall* inform-ation. In principle, these same processes are also a part of memory.

Getting things you want to remember into the files (acquiring)

Temporary memory

So we have our filing cabinet ready to be filled up with more new memories. How do we get them in there? There are a few steps in this process.

First we *pay attention* to the information—we need to be awake and alert here—and it goes into a small temporary store, often referred to as **working memory**. You could think of this temporary memory as your in-tray, which you keep on top of your filing cabinet. The working memory system temporarily holds and processes small amounts of information. Later the information goes into more enduring storage.

When temporary memory is used to repeat information for immediate use, this is how it works:

- You *do not process* or manipulate the information that goes into it. The information gets in and sits in your in-tray without being checked over or organised in any way.
- It can only hold a small amount of information at one time. Your in-tray is small and has a very *limited capacity*. It can hold five to eight items at one time.
- The next information that you put into this temporary store will wipe out what was in it before. Each time new items are placed in your in-tray, the previous items are moved out to make more room.

Now, have a go at using this temporary memory process so that you can test out what we're talking about.

Read the following telephone number slowly. When you have finished reading it, stop, and say the telephone number to your-self: 9412 5738.

Now, here's some more information to put into your in-tray. You are at a meeting and someone introduces himself to you. He says, 'Hi, I'm Anton Pillay.' Now repeat the name to yourself.

After you put the name 'Anton Pillay' into your in-tray, you probably found it hard to remember the phone number that you've just repeated. If so, it was moved out, to make more room. This type of memory is good for remembering a phone number long enough to dial it, but doesn't last long enough for you to dial the same number again half an hour later (or even five minutes later!).

Enduring memory

Let's say that you want to save that phone number for later use, but you don't have a pen and paper handy to write it down or your phone at hand to type it straight in. Or perhaps you want to remember Anton Pillay's name because you are likely to meet him again. To remember these bits of information later, you will have to move them from your in-tray into more durable storage, inside your filing cabinet.

To make the information more durable you will have to *process or manipulate* it in some way. These manipulations can happen without you being aware of it, but more often you do them intentionally. For example, you might repeat a number a few times or divide it into two or more sections to be remembered separately; you might repeat a name a few times, concentrate on its spelling or think how it is similar to the name of a person that you know very well. People sometimes use quite complex reminders which have personal significance.

I will always remember the phone number for our local take-away pizza shop. The first digits are the local dialling code, and the last four digits are 1956, the year that the Olympics were in my home town—Melbourne!
Jack, 32

When it is a name which is likely to be very important for me to recall accurately, I consciously change the way I am standing or sitting when I hear the name, repeat the name after I have left the person and as soon as possible find a pen and paper to record it.

Delys, when she was in her sixties

At other times, people acquire or collect new memories without realising it until they recall them later. This could happen when you are looking for your keys, for example. When you put the keys down, you didn't try to remember where you put them. However, when it comes to finding them later, most times you will remember without too much active recalling where you put them.

Whether new information gets in intentionally or not, it still goes through the same basic processing. It's just that sometimes you don't realise the process is occurring. You pay attention to something, it goes into your temporary memory in-tray and, from there, it is processed for the more durable storage files within your memory filing cabinet.

Scientists believe that information can be more difficult to get out of a memory file later on if it has not been processed in a meaningful and well-organised way. For instance, if you shove something into your filing cabinet in a rush, without paying attention and stopping to think about which file it should be put in, it can be difficult to find again later. If, on the other hand, you classify it, label it, and put it into a mental folder that contains other similar files, it should be much easier to locate later on.

There are many different 'filing tabs' that we use in our filing cabinet—files can be organised by what they look, sound, smell, taste or feel like. Memories that we have 'filed' and stored previously can be utilised so that we don't have to start from scratch every time we add new memories. We can build on prior memories and this helps with forming new memories. We might group files according to context—family, work, hobbies and so on. This idea is important when we think of learning and memory strategies, topics that we will return to in Chapters 6 and 7.

Take the time now to do some memory processing. Imagine you are going shopping and you want to buy nine items. Of course, most of us would use a shopping list to take the load off our memory, but for now, have a go at putting this information into your memory storage for later use. Spend a few moments working on the list below. Later you can check how successful you were!

Milk
Soap
Apples
Bananas
Yoghurt
Shampoo
Lemons
Cheese
Toothpaste

Having a good safe filing cabinet (storing)

This more enduring storage that we've been talking about is your true filing cabinet. It's where all kinds and any amounts of memories can be stored. Some are very emotional, some sad, some happy. You will store things that you've seen, heard, smelled, tasted or touched. Things in here can be very organised, or a complete mess of disorganised data (like a badly organised pantry!).

You can put as much information as you like into these files—there is no known limit to the amount of information that can go into memory storage. Your filing cabinet is bottomless. You can store information here for very long periods of time—sometimes for over 90 years!

Recent memory storage

Recent memories are those from this morning, yesterday and last week. What did you have for dinner last night? What happened in the television serial last Sunday? What was that telephone message earlier today? Recent memories are still undergoing consolidation processing and they are the ones that many of us complain about forgetting.

Lifetime memory storage

Over time, we build up a vast array of more durable memories. What we hold in lifetime memory storage, and the way we organise it, is different for each person. You can store:

- **Personal memories** from your own life history that contribute to your beliefs and your behaviour.
- Memories of **familiar places,** such as special landscapes, towns, parks, supermarkets—and the way to get around them.
- Memories of **procedures,** or knowledge of how to do things. Your store of procedures will include the activities that you have learned well and practised regularly during your life, like driving, typing, tying your shoelaces, making a sauce, etc. When you first learn these procedures it takes a lot of conscious effort, but now that you know them well, they seem automatic and it doesn't feel like you use your memory when you do them.
- Information about your **area of expertise** at work or at home. For example, you might remember and know a lot about computer software programs, accounting, teaching, cooking or gardening.
- **General knowledge** information that comes in handy for games such as Trivial Pursuit and quiz shows, and answering questions from your grandchildren!
- You also store **conceptual knowledge** and general rules that you have accumulated over time—for example, arithmetical concepts (addition, subtraction, etc.) or different shapes (round, square,

etc.), or knowledge that the earth is round and you won't fall off because of gravity.

What are some of the lifetime memories that are occupying many files in your filing cabinet? What are in some of your special skills files, your areas of expertise files? What files do you have of procedures that have become so automatic you do not have to actively think about the steps involved?

Getting things out when you need to use them (recalling)

There comes a time when you want to get memories out again, and sometimes quickly. This process is often called **recall**. Sometimes recall is for exact detail—for example, 'What is the French word for clock?' or 'What is her name?' But even when we remember a word, a name, or a song, we 'flavour' it with a meaning which is special for us as individuals. Some may remember a classroom scene when they recall words learned in language classes, or who they were once with as they sang a particular song.

What we recall from our memory files is usually quite selective, and it is not always a replica or mirror image of what went in. Even the most accurate recall will not be as exact a 'copy' as if we were pulling out the original document or the original sound or smell which was filed in our memory storage. We re-interpret, build up again or even redesign the information in the smallest or the grandest way when we bring the 'stuff' we want to remember out of storage.

But how can you say that was what Dad told us? I was there at the time and I didn't hear him say it like that!
Robert, 51, to Susan, 48

Our beliefs, our values, our perceptions not only affect what we select to put into storage; they also influence what we actually choose to remember. If Susan wants to influence her recollections because of how she values Robert, she will challenge her own memory and maybe reconstruct her perception of how her father spoke.

> 'Memory is a net; one finds it full of fish when he takes it from the brook; but a dozen miles of water have run through it without sticking.'
>
> Oliver W. Holmes Sr, 1858

Recall processes

Sometimes your filing cabinet falls open automatically and presents you with an 'uncalled-for' memory. This often happens because of **association**, and associations are often triggered by smell.

I was amazed to suddenly recall an event, out of the blue it seemed, when I must have been about eight years of age: my father was watching me drive the Caterpillar tractor, for the very first time on my own around the yard. I could see him with the pigpen yards behind him and even smell the pigs! He was coming over to the tractor. I could see the control panel very clearly. Then I heard him saying loudly, 'Pull that lever down, John.' It was so clear. What brought this into my mind just then? I know: I was driving past a farm and the smell of pigs was so strong!
John, 60

Smell can be overwhelmingly nostalgic because it triggers powerful images and emotions before we have time to edit them.

Airports smell the same everywhere for me. The smell used to make me feel dread because I was leaving the family for work, but now that I'm retired it makes me excited for holidays!
Devika, 66

When we give perfume to someone, we give them liquid memory. Kipling was right: 'Smells are surer than sights and sounds to make your heart strings crack.'[1]

Memories can also be associated with particular times of the year.

Each Christmas when I open the Christmas tree decorations box, memories come flooding back to me of past Christmas times. Each decoration has a story that goes with it, especially the handmade ones.
Elizabeth, 45

I well remember so much about Christmas days when we were young, competing with my brothers for how many threepences were in the Christmas pudding, opening the Christmas stocking before anyone else was awake, helping to cook the Christmas dinner in the heat of a Western Australian summer day, preparing the Christmas tree and opening the box of decorations from so many years before.
Delys, when she was in her sixties

I have my saddest times when I remember some of the events which occurred around Christmas Day—of arguments over who should prepare certain foods, of unwelcome family announcements, of people who have died and aren't with us anymore, of people who have preferred to share Christmas with others . . . I am starting to dread the 25th of December.
Carlos, 75

Unprompted memories can also occur by **recognition**. You may be watching a film, and realise that you've seen it before. You might not remember someone's name when you see them at a wedding, but you may recognise it when you see it on the list of names for the seating arrangement. You might see a photo of a landscape and remember an event of your childhood or a holiday.

Free recall occurs when you want to remember something, and go searching through your memory storage files to find it—the author of the book you are reading, the joke your friend told you last week, the name of the wine you had last night, the time you are to be picked up. You might have a word on the tip of your tongue, but no matter how hard you try, you can't recall it. What was her name? What is the word for the yellow spice powder that is used to flavour many curries?

When we learn something new, we usually draw on free recall. You might like to use free recall to have a go at remembering that nine-item shopping list that you read earlier. Which items can you recall now? When you've reached your limit, go back a few pages and check what they were!

The ability to **reminisce**, which contributes to the life quality of many people, is dependent on the ability to use free recall from memory storage for past events. Have a go at some free recall from your past and indulge in some reminiscence! Think back to an experience from your school days—for example, making a special friend, the sound of a particular teacher or a sports event. Remember it in as much detail as possible. For example, what was the name of the school? How old were you? Who else was there? Where were you sitting or standing? What were you wearing? What year did it happen in?

Thinking about this experience entails recall of information that was put in your lifetime memory storage a long time ago. You may find some details easier to recall than others, and if the recall is repeated some hours later, more details may emerge.

We often try to promote free recall when we use intention to remember. This type of memory is sometimes called **prospective memory** and it is important in everyday life. How often do we say, 'I must remember to remember that' or 'I mustn't forget that'. Later on, we have to recall what it was that we told ourselves to remember. It might be to take some medication, to take the cake out of the oven in 40 minutes, or to go to the hairdresser next Thursday at 3 p.m. But it can be very frustrating at times. Remembering to remember is complex—you need to plan to remember what you want to do later, retrieve the memory at the appropriate time, and then do what you had planned to do!

Recall can be made easier if we use other information or a special cue to trigger the memory. This is called **cued recall**. If you couldn't find your wallet, a cue that you might use would be to think, 'Where did I have my wallet last?' If you meet up with a man in the street, but can't remember his name, you can sometimes cue your memory by thinking about the context that you usually see him in. Is he someone from the sports club, from work or from your street? What sort of cues do you use to trigger memories? Have you ever cued your memory to help find something you have mislaid?

For many people, photos are especially important visual cues for past memories.

If I came home and saw my house on fire, the first thing I would try to get out would be my photo negatives. My photos are my personal history. I'd hate to be without them.
Len, 68

We will return to the idea of cued recall in more detail when we discuss memory strategies in Chapter 6.

There are times when we recall information from storage without realising it. For example, many of the steps involved in playing the piano, riding a bicycle, driving a car, cooking, or setting the table are procedures which have become automatic.

I'm home with my first baby, and constantly feel that I'm on a 'steep learning curve' when it comes to being a parent. I often catch myself saying, 'How do you know how to do that, Mum?' And she replies, 'I don't know really—I've just always done it that way.' Everything seems so easy for her, in comparison to my fumbling fingers. She seems to put nappies on without thinking, and makes baby bathing look so easy.
Monica, 31

Of course we don't need to remember everything, and forgetting is a vital aspect of memory. If we didn't forget information, the system would become overloaded. It is normal to forget information that is no longer relevant. We don't need to remember where we parked our car when we went to the supermarket three weeks ago, but we do want to remember where we parked it today! As noted by prominent memory theorists:

> A properly functioning memory system must be as good at forgetting as it is at remembering.[2]

We are constantly using different memory processes. Our memory filing cabinet is almost never shut. Sometimes remembering works well for us, at other times we notice lapses. Memory is dynamic. There are constant fluctuations in all of our memory processes—in getting information in, storing it and getting what we want out. In the following chapters we will explore some of the factors that can enhance the dynamics of our memory across the years of our life.

Key points   HOW MEMORY WORKS

- Memory is not a single 'thing'. At the simplest level, it involves:
  - *acquiring*: putting new information into temporary memory and more enduring memory
  - *storing*: according to when stored and type of memory
  - *recalling*: getting the information out again, by association, recognition, and free and cued recall.
- Memories are selective and are reconstructed; they are not exact replicas of experience.
- Forgetting is important—we don't need to remember everything.
- Memory is dynamic, and influenced by many factors.

CHAPTER 2

How memory changes as we get older

I don't have a memory, I have a forgettery!
Frank, 78

Why can I remember things from the past, but not what happened yesterday?
Jenny, 69

A few years ago I went to introduce my boss to someone at work and his name wouldn't come to me. I was so embarrassed.
Glenn, 58

I forget where I put things. The other day I was looking for my pen and I eventually found it in my shirt pocket, where I had put it earlier in the day.
Tim, 81

As we get older, we often notice changes in our memory. We might have problems remembering names and particular words, things that have happened recently, where we've put something, dates of appointments coming up, or what we were planning to do.

I go into a room to get something, and when I get into the room I think, 'What did I come in here to get?' This happens so often now that I jokingly refer to it as my problem with 'the hereafter'!
Ivan, 85

If we experience these problems as a younger person, we tend to blame them on lack of effort or not paying enough attention. As we get older, and experience the same memory lapses, we begin to wonder about our actual memory ability, and become concerned. We might start thinking, 'Could it be Alzheimer's?'

I am worried that I have early Alzheimer's. Recalling people's names has always been bad but now it's worse. I can't find the right word . . . you know that thing . . . when I'm saying things I know the word and then it will just go.
Ratna, 70

My father is 54 years old, and is one of the most fit and healthy people I know. He migrated to Australia some 30 years ago, with no knowledge of the English language and maybe fourth-grade education. Now he works for one of the largest retail organisations in Australia, travelling around the state, training others in his area of expertise. He is very easy-going and very social, but there is one thing that seems to worry him at times—his memory. He worries about it because his mother had Alzheimer's disease before she died five or six years ago. The things he says he forgets are names, phone numbers, dates and sometimes things that family members have told him in passing. I'm 25 years old and have the same forgetfulness—if I don't write things down, I might as well have never been told. My father is also partially deaf in one ear, so chances are he may not have even heard something that he thinks he has forgotten. And, while his grasp of the English language is very good, he sometimes misses things if a person speaks too quickly, or uses uncommon words or has a thick or unusual accent. He leads a full and busy life and has many things on his mind at any time—one would expect to forget the things he forgets! But when

I tell him this it serves only to ease his mind until the next time he can't remember something that I told him. And then what overpowers him is that his mother died of Alzheimer's disease, and that he can't remember something.
Ellen, 25

Dementia is often portrayed as an inevitable consequence of ageing in our community. The media continues to emphasise abnormal and negative aspects of ageing, which has a powerful influence on society attitudes. We are regularly exposed to portrayals of public figures experiencing memory loss and dementia, and because more people than ever before are living into their eighties and nineties, we are now more likely to have first-hand experience of someone with dementia.

For many of us, the possibility of developing dementia is one of the greatest fears of growing old. After all, memory is self. Fortunately, dementia is not a part of normal ageing: less than 1 per cent of people under 65 have Alzheimer's disease, and in the 65–75 age range the figure is still less than 5 per cent. The percentage does rise with increasing age—to around 11 per cent for those aged 80–84, and 18 per cent for those aged 85–89—but still, the vast majority of older adults do not develop dementia.[1]

The current outlook on memory and ageing

In the previous chapter, different memory processes were outlined. Only some of these have been shown to change as people get older. Some memory processes are found not to be affected at all, and some can improve, so the picture is certainly not one of dramatic, inevitable and accelerating decline.

For many people, changes in particular memory processes happen so gradually that they are not thought of as a problem. For others, the changes are only obvious in situations where they are required to push their memory abilities to the limit.

The bulk of past memory research involved stretching people's memory to the utmost, and has resulted in an unnecessarily pessimistic view of the effect of old age on memory. Typical research compared the performance of young and old people on the same memory tests. Older people may have performed worse on testing, not because of their age, but due to comparative differences in their health, senses such as hearing, or level of education. Younger people could have been advantaged by familiarity with the type of tests used and the environment in which they were conducted. Moreover, many of the tests used measured speed of response, rather than actual memory ability. It is well known that younger people process information more rapidly than older people.[2] They get new information into their storage files faster. We have all had the experience of observing how quickly five-year-olds learn how to use new technology! Finally, we should not forget that motivated older people can use life skills and adapt their learning by being very strategic (see Chapter 6), using their developed wisdom to manage effective learning.

Memory abilities at any age will be different for one person compared to another. At your book club you might notice that one person is able to remember all the details from a book they have just read, whereas another person might have difficulty recalling such details. There are many factors found to enhance this variability between people of the same age, and even in the same individual from day to day. These health, attitude and lifestyle factors will be discussed in Chapter 3.

Which memory processes change as we get older?

Research has described the effect of getting older on attention processes, the ability to get new information into storage, the time that it takes to learn new things, and the 'tip of the tongue' experience. It is often a combination of these changes, together with aspects of our health and the way we live our lives, that can make our memory more unreliable as we get older.

Attention

Research has shown that as we get older we can experience change in our ability to pay attention, and our ability to ignore distractions. These aspects of paying attention are part of 'working memory' as outlined in Chapter 1.

Some studies have shown that older people cannot focus attention on as much information at the same time as younger people. Furthermore, older people can find it difficult to shift their attention back and forth between two tasks.[3] This may mean that it is harder to follow two conversations at the same time, or it may be more difficult to do several things at once—for instance, reading a book with music playing in the background and at the same time remembering not to let the casserole in the oven overcook.

Where did I put my phone? I may have three things on my mind—put the washing on, reply to that email and where is my phone? When I multi-task now I'm not as good as I was 10 years ago. I worry that my memory is going.
Jillian, 62

Older people have also been shown to have more difficulty resisting distraction.[4] Distraction can be internal or external. A common internal distraction is when we are thinking about something else or registering pain, and find that we have let our mind wander. A common external distraction is the phone. You are busy doing something when your phone rings. You answer your phone, and later find it hard to remember what you were doing before the phone interrupted you.

I can't remember what my friends tell me on the phone because they ring me when I'm at work and I'm distracted and feel interrupted.
Leona, 59

In these situations we have trouble getting new information into our storage files, because we are finding it harder to pay attention to it. Many 'memory' lapses are not so much memory, but attentional lapses.

Of course, changes in our senses with ageing can have an additional impact on our ability to focus attention.[5] For example, if we have hearing or visual impairment, we allocate more attention to trying to hear or see incoming information. This means we have less attentional resources to dedicate to forming a memory of what is around us.[6]

My wife says I forget what she has told me. She might mention something once and if I don't write it down, or she doesn't remind me again, it might get lost. I wonder if my hearing problem has something to do with this. I sometimes find it hard to hear what she is saying, especially if there is background noise from the TV or radio.
Eric, 86

The ability to remember new things

As we have discussed in the previous chapter, remembering something new involves the processes of acquiring, storing and recalling. Research has shown that our acquiring and recalling processes can be affected as we get older.[7]

As we age, we have more difficulty on tests that involve remembering things that we have just seen or heard. Older people have been found to be less likely than younger people to use memory strategies, such as the way they organise their thinking, what they associate with information, or how they 'see' things in their mind, to help them to acquire or recall new information. The information may be stored, but unless it is well filed, it is hard to get at when needed. When you put a library book back on the wrong shelf, or the balsamic vinegar bottle in with the wine bottles, it is as good as missing.

Researchers have begun to ask why is it that many older people don't spontaneously make use of strategies to help them remember new things. Could it be that older people were never taught to use these strategies? Many older people of today were taught to rely on rote learning, while school education has more recently focused on using meaning and association to remember. Or could it be that using such strategies is more difficult for older people because they are slower to process information or have more difficulty with 'working memory' processes? Information is often presented rapidly, and older people may need more time than when they were younger to organise it into the proper files in their filing system.

The time that it takes to remember things

Mastering something new takes more time as we age. Extra time may be required for practice and review in order to acquire new skills, such as speaking a new language, cooking a new recipe, or managing the intricacies of new technologies.

As a 56-year-old mature-age university student, I am noticing that I need to go over information many more times when preparing for exams than I did when I studied in my twenties.
Chan, 56

I am learning Japanese. I can learn the information, but it takes a lot longer than it would have taken me when I was younger. I have to put in more effort. I write organised notes and read over them several times. I can't rely on memory; I have to rely on methodology. When I'm learning new words, I need to build bridges. Once the bridges are there, I can recall the information. For example, I spent hours trying to learn the word 'kudasai' in Japanese. It just wouldn't come, every time I tried to recall it. So I associated it with the word 'cuckoo', and this gave me the first sound of the word. Now I can easily remember it.
Patrick, 71

When we get older it can take longer to get information out of the storage files, as well as into them.[8] This is most evident when an immediate response to something is required. You might have difficulty recalling someone's name when you meet them in the street, or you might draw a blank when someone asks you what you did last weekend, but you can often remember the information later. The impact of this slowing is not so obvious in responding to familiar or more routine requests for quick memory recall. If an activity is second nature, it can be performed without a great deal of mental effort and the 'normal' slowing associated with older age doesn't affect it so much.

The 'tip of the tongue' experience

'Memory is often not so much lost as hard to find.'[9]

Most of us have had the 'tip of the tongue' experience. We say, 'What is that word . . . I know it, but I can't recall it', or, 'What is that person's name—I know it so well, but it won't come to me.' Whenever we want to remember something, we review the contents of the files in our filing cabinet. People of all ages can experience 'blocking'—when a search for particular information is not successful.

I'm having a brain-freeze: I know it's there, but it won't come up!
Yanina, 54

A 'tip of the tongue' experience occurs when our search process gets close to the word or name, but we cannot 'locate' the file for it. The word that we want to say is typically a word we don't use frequently. Difficulty finding a word is different to recalling something that we have just learned. It involves sorting through old storage files for a memory that has been there for a long time, and that we know very well is in there for us to find.

When I went to buy my meat at the butcher's yesterday, I had a blank for the word 'skewers'. I covered it up by asking for 'the chicken on sticks', and thankfully the butcher knew what I was talking about.
Steve, 73

Research has shown that we experience the 'tip of the tongue' problem more often as we get older.[10] Some researchers suggest that this is because our storage files get larger as we get older and we have more information to search through. Names of people are a common example. Perhaps, after a lifetime of meeting people, it becomes more difficult to pluck out one particular name, especially if it is similar to many other names that we have stored in our files.

I wish my brain was as fast as my computer. I find that my brain's 'search engine' is much slower now that I'm older.
Rico, 57

Another theory relates to the context that we are in when we are doing a memory search of our files. It is much easier to identify and name someone when we always see them in the same place or at predictable times. But we all know how difficult it can be to remember someone's name when we meet up with them unexpectedly in a new context. As we get older, it seems we become more dependent on contextual cues.

I was at my local shopping centre last week and I walked past a woman who smiled at me and looked familiar but I couldn't work out where I knew her from. Later I sifted through in my mind all the places where I meet people. Was it through work, through the kids? The next day it suddenly came to me: I had met her when my daughter was at primary school 15 years ago—her daughter's name is Francesca and she is Fay!
Naya, 56

So as we get older our memory is influenced by our ability to attend, the context (the where and when), needing more time to process our files, and the ever increasing amount of information stored in our files (some of which we may not have organised very well!).

Which areas of memory will not be affected by age?

Research suggests our lifetime memories are less sensitive to the ageing process.[11] The various forms of lifetime memories were described in the previous chapter: personal memories; information about your area of expertise at work or at home; memories of familiar places; memories of procedures such as riding a bike or playing a musical instrument; general knowledge and conceptual knowledge. We might not be able to recall some specific details, such as the exact dates of past memories, but in general our lifetime memories are very enduring. They also keep accumulating throughout our lives. We continue to broaden our knowledge through reading, socialising, listening to the radio, watching television or participating in education programs.

Our strong lifetime memories help to give us a sense of self and are part of what is often referred to as the wisdom that comes with getting older. The memories and stories of older adults are often highly valued contributions to family and community memory. In some cultures certain older people are assigned elder status, and their memories are accorded great respect. With age and increasing experience, older adults are often called on to mentor younger people as their expertise deepens. Many leaders are older adults, who draw on past experiences and learnings to resolve conflicts by seeing problems from multiple perspectives.

Many older adults take the time to write down their lifetime memories to ensure that the memories will not be lost, and will be passed on to others over time. Older people who spend a lot of time recalling past life experiences can be negatively judged by family and friends as 'living in the past'. Yet some people use such reminiscences to work on 'unfinished business', which may often be emotive or painful. Reminiscence can also be therapeutic in a group setting, where older people share enduring memories of life experiences and are valued for their diverse range of experience. When we reminisce and bring our older memories back, we promote our sense of self and, in turn, we strengthen our sense of family and community.

Memory-wise ageing

It's important to be positive about the many continued strengths we have in our memory processes as we get older, but at the same time we need to acknowledge that it is likely that we will experience some age-related changes in our memory. Our brain is like any other part of our body: it can change as we get older, and it can be hard to accept this change when it occurs. Alterations in the efficiency of our memory processes can give us a sense of loss and make us feel frustrated and sad at times. Just like any other aspect of ageing, we can be proactive, and work on ways to enhance brain health and memory as we get older. The importance of nurturing our memory through addressing aspects of our health, lifestyle and attitude is addressed in the following chapter. The latest findings on optimising brain health are described in Chapter 5, and practical everyday memory strategies to get the most out of memory are suggested in Chapters 6 and 7.

Key points   HOW MEMORY CHANGES AS WE GET OLDER

- As we get older, we often notice changes in our memory.
- Dementia, such as Alzheimer's disease, is not a part of normal ageing, and the vast majority of older adults will not develop dementia.

- Knowledge about how memory changes as we get older is a lot more positive than in the past. Memory change with healthy ageing doesn't interfere with everyday life in a dramatic way.
- Everyone is different, and the effect on memory of getting older is different for each person.
- Memory researchers have described age-related changes in attention processes, acquiring and recalling new information, the time that it takes to learn new things, and the 'tip of the tongue' experience.
- Lifetime memories continue to accumulate as we get older, and our community benefits from the experience and wisdom of older adults.

CHAPTER 3

What else affects memory? Health, attitude, lifestyle

At any age, our memory abilities will be sensitive to what is going on in our lives. In this chapter, people's stories will be used to illustrate the often complex interaction of physical and emotional factors that can affect memory. Some factors are beyond our control—for example, a stroke can cause permanent changes to our ability to remember. However, there are choices we can make, to do with our health, lifestyle and attitude towards remembering, that will help us get more out of our memory.

How 'healthy' your memory is depends quite a bit on how healthy you are. Many of us notice fluctuations in our ability to remember when we experience changes in our physical wellbeing—when we are hospitalised, after a general anaesthetic, or even when experiencing a severe cold.

We can find that our ability to remember is worse when we are experiencing emotional stresses; during menopause; during bereavement; or when we're leading a very active social life combined with a heavy workload and complex relationships. Taking steps to deal with stress or excessive busyness can improve our remembering.

Our attitudes towards our memory are important. Negative expectations can become a self-fulfilling prophecy. If we think we have no control over our memory abilities, we may never take action.

The following four stories show how aspects of our health, lifestyle and attitude towards remembering can influence memory. Each story is followed by an analysis and some suggestions for action to enhance memory.

STORY 1 **Barbara, 72**

'I panic when I forget something—I'm scared that I've got early signs of Alzheimer's.'

I ended up in tears yesterday. I had dashed up to the local shopping centre in the morning to buy a present for my little grandson's birthday party that afternoon. Of course, I had left it to the last minute, and I only had half an hour to buy the gift. As I parked the car, I was running through possible gift ideas in my head. I found a present fairly quickly, rushed back out to the car park, and realised straight away that I couldn't remember where I had parked my car. I felt my heart beating in my chest and my hands started to shake. 'Oh no!' I thought, 'Mum did this—I'm sure she did this too, at about the same age as me, and she ended up with dementia.' I had to get home. I told myself to stop thinking about Mum and I did everything I could to calm myself down. I walked to all the usual places that I park my car, and eventually I found it.

Why is it that I can remember things from my past in so much detail, but I can't remember where I parked my car half an hour ago? It's not just the car. For several months now I've noticed that I forget things. I'll go into a room at home, and think, 'What was I supposed to be doing?', or I'll be talking to someone, and lose the word that I want to say. I feel like I'm always forgetting where I put my reading glasses. I panic when I forget something—I'm scared that I've got early signs of Alzheimer's. I feel so disorganised and stupid and I keep telling myself how bad my memory is.

I find myself saying 'no' more and more when I'm asked to go out with friends and family. I'm worried that I'll forget something in their company; it's easier to just stay at home. I feel better doing things that I can still do well, like sewing my patchwork quilts and baking treats for the grandchildren. I'm going to have to get in the car again tomorrow though—I need to go to the doctor to get a script for medication for my back. I've had pain in my back for many years now, but the pain always seems worse when I worry more, and yesterday it felt overwhelming.

Barbara's situation is all too common. There are many factors that influence how her memory works for her.

Age

Barbara is 72, and she describes some of the changes in remembering that many older people experience. Barbara has trouble getting new things into memory storage, and getting stored information—like particular words—out quickly. She also says her memory for the past and for procedures like sewing and baking is okay. This pattern of strengths and inefficiencies in memory fits well with what is known about age-related memory change.

Health (anxiety, chronic pain)

Barbara describes feelings of worry and fear, and she notices her heart beating in her chest and her hands starting to shake when she panics. These are all common features of **anxiety** and panic. A sense of panic can also be accompanied by breathing difficulties, such as very rapid breathing or feeling breathless without exertion. Other anxiety symptoms include feeling restless, irritable and becoming easily tired. Muscular tension and problems with concentration and sleep are also common. Severe anxiety can have a negative effect on attention and memory.[1] If feelings of anxiety, worry and/or fear persist over several weeks and start to affect your ability to function, it is important to see your doctor to discuss appropriate treatment. This may involve referral to a psychiatrist or psychologist to work on ways to manage the symptoms of anxiety.

Anxiety about memory loss can lead to an actual worsening of memory function, which can be thought of as a **memory–anxiety spiral**. Barbara is anxious about her memory, so she notices every time she has a memory lapse. Each time she 'forgets' something, it gives her more support for her theory about losing her memory due to early Alzheimer's disease, so she gets more anxious; anxiety probably lowers her ability to concentrate and pay attention, so she seems to be getting more forgetful, and so more anxious.

Barbara's difficulty with remembering may be further exaggerated at the moment because of **chronic pain** in her back. When someone has constant pain, it often affects their ability to concentrate and pay attention. This may be directly related to the pain, but could also be due to possible side-effects of particular pain medications, or associated disturbance to sleep and/or mood. Barbara may not, in fact, be 'forgetting' information—it may not be getting into her memory storage in the first place, because she has not paid adequate attention to it.

Attitude (negative expectation, poor self-confidence)

Barbara has developed **negative expectations** about her memory. After some months of difficulty with remembering, she now does not expect to remember well, and says she feels 'stupid'. She has little self-confidence when it comes to remembering, and subsequently little motivation to remember. She has started to avoid situations where she will have to use her memory. She withdraws from social interactions, and spends more time alone at home. She now believes that her memory is poor. Sometimes, people's beliefs about themselves can become self-fulfilling prophecies. 'I think therefore I am' is a well-known quote, and applied to memory, it could be rephrased as, 'I think I will forget, so I do forget.'

Researchers have shown that whether we assess ourselves as competent, or not, is one of the most important aspects of memory functioning in older adults. Feeling **under-confiden**t about memory can lead to a worsening in performance on memory tests.[2] If you doubt your memory ability, you most likely tend to avoid situations where you will need to use your memory. You can then easily lose confidence and make your memory worse than it actually is. You don't lack ability—you lack self-confidence in using it!

If Barbara continues to believe that she does not have a good memory, then she will feel her memory is worse than it actually is. It won't help her to 'catastrophise' and tell herself that she is 'always forgetting' things and that her memory is bad.

Lifestyle (social connections, supportive memory strategies, new learning activities)

Barbara has been less likely to socialise with friends and family recently, but maintaining her **social connections** could help her to feel more positive about herself and her capabilities. Feeling good about oneself is definitely a good thing for memory function. When Barbara values herself, she will achieve a personal affirmation of her ability.

If Barbara uses specific **strategies to support her memory**, she may feel more confident about attending social activities. She can use reminder notes to remember the details of any upcoming events, such as the time and date, location, directions for how to get there and things she needs to take with her. See Chapter 6 for more information about everyday memory strategies.

Barbara says she has been spending most of her time doing familiar activities such as baking and sewing. She has been avoiding doing anything that might lead to a memory failure, which means she is less likely to challenge herself with new experiences. Researchers have shown that if we take part in **activities that involve new learning**, changes can occur in parts of the brain that support the learning process.[3] In addition, when we experience success with learning something new, we often start to feel more confident about our memory.

Barbara could introduce some social activities into her routine that involve new learning, such as asking an older grandchild to teach her how to use a new phone app or learning a new craft technique with a group of friends. These activities would provide the benefits of both socialising and mental stimulation. Of course, Barbara could still complete many pastimes that involve new learning on her own, such as listening to a complex discussion on the radio, or mastering a new cooking technique.

Barbara will need to work out how she can fit these activities into her life. It will be best if she spends time on new activities when her back pain is manageable and she feels most energised and less anxious. She may need to make a conscious effort to reduce any possible distractions when learning new information, and work in short bursts with regular relaxation breaks.

Barbara would benefit from:

- knowing about expected memory changes that can occur with normal ageing
- receiving reassurance that in her case she does not have the type of memory difficulties that are suggestive of the early stages of Alzheimer's disease (see Chapter 8)
- identifying some of the factors that she can control which may be exaggerating her memory problem at the moment
- discussing her feelings of anxiety and panic with her doctor; this may lead to referral to a psychiatrist or psychologist for further assessment and treatment
- identifying and using appropriate pain management strategies, with assistance from her doctor and possible referral to a multi-disciplinary pain clinic, where she could see specialists in pain medicine and other health professionals including psychologists and physiotherapists
- staying socially connected
- taking part in regular new learning activities.

STORY 2 **Martin, 41**

'I feel like I'm in a fog and I can't remember information when I need it.'

After our son was born, we bought a bigger house and over-extended ourselves financially. It was getting harder and harder to find the money for the mortgage, so a few months ago I took on a new role at work with better pay. I expected the job to be demanding, but I didn't realise how overwhelmed and tired I would feel. I'm now working 12-hour days and I often do work at home in the evenings or on the weekend. I'm working on several new challenging projects. I have to learn new work procedures and I'm meeting new people each week. I keep forgetting the names of my work colleagues, even though I've been told their names several times. Information just doesn't seem to get in and I start to panic. I used to be able to remember things that we discussed in team meetings without taking notes, but now my head feels heavy and I get distracted easily. I've forgotten what my manager has asked me to do twice now. I feel like I'm in a fog and I can't recall information when I need it.

My memory is unreliable at home, too. Last week I forgot to go to my son's music concert at school. I felt so bad and he was so upset. My family life is suffering and so is my relationship with my wife. I'm hardly ever home for dinner—instead I grab take-away food and eat it in the car on the way home. My wife goes to bed before me, and I end up hitting the alcohol pretty hard at night. I feel so 'on edge' all the time I drink alcohol to help me unwind. My wife complains that she hardly ever sees me now. I'm missing seeing friends and exercising too. I used to train at the gym three times a week and ride my bike with some mates on Sunday mornings, but that all stopped when I started the new job. This lack of exercise is getting to me, because I know that when I'm fit, my energy levels are better, and I get less tired.

Many people in Martin's situation would begin to notice that their memory is not as reliable as it usually is. There are several aspects of Martin's life that he can alter if he wants to get more out of his memory.

Lifestyle (stress, workload, fatigue, relationship problems)

Martin has noticed significant changes in his memory since he started his new job. His heavy workload seems to be leading to **stress** and **fatigue**. Prolonged stress and elevations in stress hormones have been shown to have an adverse effect on memory performance.[4] Everyday memory lapses are often related to doing too much, especially doing too many things at once. Add exhaustion and stress to this, and you've got a pretty mean combination as far as memory goes! This combination could have a direct effect on Martin's ability to concentrate and pay attention. He has probably not 'forgotten' his work colleagues' names or that he was meant to go to his son's school concert—he probably never got these bits of information into his memory filing cabinet in the first place, because he wasn't paying attention to them at the time.

Martin is concerned about his relationship with his wife. This concern could also be reducing his ability to concentrate. The stress of **relationship difficulties** can often occupy our minds, and mean that it is difficult to take new information in.

Health (physical exercise, diet, alcohol)

The healthier you are, the better your memory will function. Martin says that when he is physically fit and participating in regular exercise, his energy level improves. If his energy level is higher, then he may be able to handle his workload and social commitments more easily. Physical exercise has been shown to have a positive effect on stress, and also on anxiety and depression.[5] With less stress and fatigue, Martin should be able to concentrate and pay attention to things around him more easily. Of course this will have a positive effect on his memory.

At the moment, Martin is not getting any regular **physical exercise**. He has given up training at the gym and cycling because of work commitments. He also seems to have given up on the idea of healthy eating, which of course is critical to good health. His **diet** would certainly not be described as 'balanced'.

Martin will need to watch his **alcohol** consumption. The current Australian National Health and Medical Research Council (NHMRC) guidelines recommend that drinking no more than two standard drinks a day reduces the lifetime risk of harm from alcohol-related disease or injury. An additional recommendation is to consume no more than four standard drinks on a single occasion to reduce the risk of alcohol-related injury arising from that occasion. A 'standard drink' is defined as a drink containing 10 grams of alcohol—for example, a small glass of wine (100 ml), a 375 ml can of mid-strength beer, or a 30 ml nip of spirits.

Our community is becoming increasingly aware of the effect of alcohol on health and on memory. It is now a legal requirement in Australia for the labels of all bottles, cans and casks of alcoholic drinks to state the approximate number of standard drinks they contain.

If alcohol consumption regularly exceeds the NHMRC guidelines, it can cause damage to areas of the brain that are needed for memory function. The direct effect of alcohol on the memory processes of heavy drinkers may be compounded by nutritional deficiencies, psychiatric disorders, traumatic brain injury, vascular disease of the brain, cirrhosis of the liver, other diseases and other drug use. Research shows that there is potential for improvement in memory abilities when people who have been dependent on alcohol cease drinking alcohol.[6]

Attitude (negative expectation and self-fulfilling prophecies)

Martin appears to have given up on his memory. He now calls himself someone with an 'unreliable' memory. He is close to telling himself that it will always be so. If he expects to have memory lapses, then he might stop trying to remember, and so get into a self-perpetuating cycle.

Martin would benefit from:

- realising that his memory ability is largely in his control, and that he can take action
- not labelling himself as someone whose memory is permanently 'unreliable', but rather as someone whose memory is being affected by the situation he is currently in
- using memory strategies as a back-up system, so that he believes his memory will be reliable. If he doesn't already use a reminder system, he would be well advised to start doing so. Whenever he is asked to attend a function or is directed to do something, he could add this information to his reminder system.

Martin should also focus on reducing his stress at work, with good time management. If he can do this, his ability to concentrate and pay attention should improve, which could have a direct effect on his ability to remember. At work he will need to prioritise jobs, and work on one at a time. He will need to make a real effort to focus on the task at hand, not to let his mind wander on to other things, to reduce any obvious distractions, and if he is interrupted while doing something, to go back to it as soon as possible afterwards.

Finally, Martin's goals should include:

- having regular relaxation breaks at work, even if they only last for 5 minutes
- focusing on his health—improving his diet, limiting his alcohol intake, and making about 30 minutes of regular daily exercise part of his life
- scheduling time with his wife and family
- taking steps to discuss his relationship concerns with his wife, and working on the damaging conflicts that are emerging between them.

STORY 3 **Voula, 55**

'I just can't concentrate . . . my memory is hopeless.'

Since Mum died last year everything has changed for me. I've gone from working in a fantastic part-time job to spending most of my time making sure Dad is okay. I didn't realise how much Mum did for him, and it's so sad that we are now facing the reality of moving Dad into residential care.

I feel like a part of me died when Mum died. The fun, happy Voula seems to have disappeared now. I don't feel like doing anything anymore. I used to enjoy going to work, but I had to give that up to be there for Mum when she was sick, and now I'm visiting Dad a few times a day to help him with his meals and running the house. I don't think I'll be able to get back into working again. My two brothers have never really helped out when it comes to our parents, and someone has to be there for Dad.

My sleep was already a problem before I lost Mum, and I was going through menopause. I kept waking up on and off during the night dripping with sweat from hot flushes. I used to be able to drop back off to sleep fairly easily then, but now I have trouble getting off to sleep, and when I wake up during the night I tend to lie awake for hours. I probably only get about three or four hours sleep a night now.

I'm tired all the time, but I have to push myself to do things for the family. My husband works full time and my son and daughter are both studying at university and still living at home, as they can't afford to move out yet. I feel like all I do is look after other people—cleaning, washing clothes, and cooking meals that I don't even feel like eating. I've been trying to fill out all the paperwork for Dad's move into the aged-care facility, but I just can't concentrate when I try. I was meant to call Dad's accountant yesterday morning, but I completely forgot. When I was at work, I was making important decisions every day, but deciding which care facility will be best for Dad is just too much for me at the moment.

I'm having trouble keeping track of everyone's movements. Yesterday my daughter snapped at me after I'd asked her for the third time whether she'd be home for dinner. My memory is hopeless and I wonder if this is related to menopause. I keep losing things. I go to use my phone, and I can't find it. I'm having mental blanks and it's like my mind won't grab information. We have a new neighbour, and I keep forgetting her name. I've almost given up on trying to learn her name. If I see her in the street, I tend to avoid talking to her now. I wouldn't have much to say to her anyway—I'm so boring these days.

Voula wonders whether her memory problem is related to menopause. While it is possible that menopause may be contributing to her difficulties, there are other aspects of Voula's current situation that are likely to be affecting her memory.

Health (menopause, sleep, depression)

Many women notice changes in their memory around the time of **menopause**, and the following chapter covers this topic in detail. While some studies have reported subtle changes in some aspects of memory during menopause, research has not revealed consistent evidence of significant memory loss directly related to menopause.[7]

Voula described difficulties with sleep over the past year, and disrupted sleep patterns are common during menopause and also with depression. During menopause, hot flushes and night-time sweats can interrupt sleep. With depression, it is common to have difficulty falling asleep and difficulty staying asleep. It is possible that Voula's sleep difficulties are contributing to her memory difficulties.

The importance of **sleep** for memory function has been highlighted in recent research.[8] Sleep has been shown to be crucial both before and after learning new information. Good-quality sleep is required to enhance the memory system's processing of incoming information, and also to promote the formation of memories during sleep. Performance on tasks that involve attention and new learning has been shown to be affected by poor sleep. Sleep loss also leads to slower speed in thinking processes. Research has demonstrated that significant sleep loss can lead to changes in areas of the brain that are important to attention and memory, and that when sleep patterns are restored to normal, there is improvement in memory function.[9]

Voula could seek advice from her doctor for improving her sleep. In addition, she could see a psychologist to work on personalised strategies.

Strategies to enhance sleep include:

- going to bed at the same time each night, and rising at the same time each morning
- limiting day-time naps to 15–20 minutes
- exercising each day, keeping more energetic workouts for the mornings and more relaxing exercise for the evenings
- limiting caffeine intake, and not drinking too many liquids in the evening, including alcohol
- avoiding big meals at night, especially spicy and sugary foods
- avoiding television, computer, tablet and phone screens close to bedtime
- establishing a calming routine before bed, and doing something relaxing.

If Voula finds herself waking during the night and worrying about something, she should make a note of it, and tell herself she can deal with it in the morning. She should then distract herself by doing something mundane, like counting or muscle relaxation.

As well as her difficulty sleeping, Voula describes other symptoms of **depression**. She has felt unhappy since her mother died several months ago, and she describes a lack of enthusiasm and initiative, with not much to look forward to. Her self-esteem appears low, and she calls herself 'boring'. She is constantly tired, her appetite has lessened, and she says she has trouble concentrating and making decisions. Voula's negative feelings have started to have an effect on her life. For example, she is less likely to socialise now. Since these symptoms have persisted for more than two weeks, it is likely that she has depression.

People who have depression often remark that their memory is poor. Of course, not all people with depression experience memory difficulties. When they do, it is usually only some aspects of memory that are problematic. When people are depressed they are usually less motivated than usual and can feel ambivalent about things that would usually interest them. This can make it difficult to learn new things, as they find it hard to focus and concentrate on new information. This can, of course, affect their ability to get new information into memory storage—the initial acquisition phase. Problems with paying attention can lead to inefficient processing of incoming information. This may explain why Voula forgot what her daughter said to her about being home for dinner, and why she forgot where she put her phone and the name of her new neighbour. Effortful memory processes, such as prospective memory, which involve remembering to remember something, can also be difficult when someone has depression. An example of this for Voula was when she forgot to call her father's accountant at a specific time. Researchers examining memory and depression have described these difficulties as memory problems associated with symptoms of depression, such as reduced motivation and inattention. Studies have also suggested that depression can affect parts of the brain that are important to memory, which can further compound memory issues during depression.[10]

If feelings of unhappiness make it difficult to function in everyday life, and these feelings persist for more than two weeks, it is important to seek medical advice. Treatment for depression can involve both medication and psychological care, and different types of depression need different approaches. With appropriate treatment, many people notice that their memory improves, along with their mood.

Lifestyle (overload)

Voula sounds exhausted. She is not sleeping well, and her days are full of family commitments. She seems to spend all of her time doing things for others—her father, her husband and her children—with little time to rest and take care of herself. Being so busy and tired would not be helping Voula's memory.

Attitude (hopelessness)

Voula says, 'My memory is hopeless.' Every time she has a memory lapse, she uses that experience to strengthen her theory that her memory is hopeless. She blames the problem on menopause, and has given up on seeking ways to help her memory. With this attitude, her memory is not likely to get any better. She seems to think that she has no direct control over how well her memory can be made to work for her.

Voula could be encouraged to develop more realistic expectations of her memory. It would help if she was more patient with herself. When she forgets something, she could stay calm and say to herself, 'There is a reason why I forgot that—I'm tired, overwhelmed and feeling flat', rather than, 'I am hopeless.' The way we react to our memory lapses is important. We need to be kind to ourselves when we are experiencing difficult times in our lives.

We don't need to remember everything, but for those important things that we do want to recall, we can use simple strategies to make us feel more confident in our memory. Voula mentioned that she keeps losing her phone. This is a common lapse related to not paying attention. Voula most likely puts her phone down while she is distracted and thinking about something else. There are several strategies that could help Voula be more mindful and pay more attention. When Voula puts her phone down, she could say in her head, or out loud: 'I am putting my phone on the kitchen bench.' She could make an effort to always put her phone in the same spot in her house or her handbag. To be totally confident that she will be able to find her phone, she could attach a location tracking device to it. Having a brightly coloured phone case could also help. Chapter 6 provides more information about useful everyday memory strategies to enhance confidence in remembering.

Voula would benefit from:

- acknowledging that there are some aspects of her life that she has the potential to control; if she works on these, she may find her memory improves
- seeing her doctor to talk about menopause, sleep and depression; this may involve referral to a psychiatrist and a psychologist for further treatment and support
- creating some time for herself by asking her brothers to help care for their father
- asking her husband and adult children to help out with household jobs such as cooking and cleaning
- making time for 30 minutes of moderate physical activity a day
- allowing time each day to do a small, simple activity that brings joy, such as a short walk in a natural setting outdoors
- being patient with herself and developing realistic expectations of her memory during this overwhelming time of her life
- using memory strategies as a 'back-up system' to get around her current difficulty with concentration and attention, which will also combat her feeling of 'hopelessness', and show her that she can and already does remember many things; Chapter 6 describes a variety of specific memory strategies.

STORY 4 **Gordon, 64**

'I thought his memory would get better after the stroke, but lately it has started to get worse.'

My husband, Gordon, had a mild stroke three years ago, just after he retired from his work as a builder. Ever since, he has had a slight problem with his memory. The specialists at the rehabilitation centre told us that this was due to the memory areas of the brain being affected in a mild way by his stroke.

He's okay when it comes to remembering things from the past. It's just remembering more recent things that he has trouble with. It has been a very subtle change, so not many other people outside the family have noticed.

Over the last three months, I've noticed that the problem with his memory has gradually got worse. When I say this to him, he says, 'It's from the stroke, and there's nothing I can do about it.' Unfortunately the stroke seems to have left him with that 'resigned to my fate' attitude. He is quite apathetic. The doctors told me that people's personalities can change in this way after a stroke.

We moved into a smaller unit about three months ago. The house that Gordon built for us as a family was getting too much for us to manage. The garden was large, and we just couldn't keep it to the standard we wanted. It was sad to leave the house that we had been in since we were married, but we just had to be practical.

A few months ago he had trouble with his throat—needing to clear it all the time and feeling an ache in his neck muscles, yet he didn't have a cold. A specialist thought his throat muscles were in strain and put him on Valium, to relax the muscles. It seems to be helping with the muscular problem, but I wonder if it has any side-effects on his memory? He seems to be less able to concentrate.

Lately, I've noticed that Gordon is asking me to repeat what I say to him quite often. I'm sure his hearing has got worse. When I think about it, it's usually things people tell him that he forgets. He also often asks me to tell him where things are around the unit. Now that we're in a smaller place, we've had to change where we keep most of our things.

I'll have to do something about this. The specialists told me he would get better with time, not worse.

Lilian

Gordon's wife has reason to feel concerned. He does have a real brain injury and a consequent memory problem due to the stroke, but the changes Lilian has observed in Gordon over the last three months are likely to be related to additional factors unrelated to his stroke. If Gordon and Lilian can be helped to identify and address these complicating factors, they will be likely to notice a positive effect on Gordon's memory.

Health (brain injury, grief, hearing impairment, side-effects of medication)

Gordon has been told that he sustained mild damage to the brain from his stroke, particularly in the areas that are needed for some aspects of memory function. The stroke has most likely caused limitations in his ability to get new information into storage, and to be able to recall it later.

There are many other causes of change to the memory areas of the brain, apart from strokes. For example, serious head injuries, particular brain tumours, and certain forms of epilepsy can alter our ability to remember. Major operations can also sometimes affect memory function. We will discuss memory loss related to dementia and Alzheimer's disease in Chapter 8. With any known **brain condition**, it is important to check continually for health, lifestyle and attitude factors that could be making the memory problem worse than it is.

Lilian also mentioned that Gordon's personality changed after the stroke. He became more apathetic. A lack of motivation, no matter what the cause, can affect remembering in a negative way. If you are not motivated to remember something, you are less likely to get it into your memory filing cabinet.

Gordon may have some **grief** issues, which are not obvious to his wife. He has suffered some real losses due to his stroke. He has also recently retired and moved from the house that he built when he and Lilian married. His retirement and the house move could be additional major losses for Gordon. Grief and adjustment to loss can affect people's ability to concentrate and pay attention, which in turn make it difficult to learn new information.

Gordon's **hearing** may be another factor that is affecting his ability to get new information into storage. If you don't hear something, then that information will not go into your temporary memory storage for processing—which means it will not get into your more enduring storage files. It is important to be aware of the effect of sensory loss on memory. Our senses of hearing, vision, smell, touch and taste are important to the processes of remembering.

When hearing is a problem, the following may help.

- Face the person when you are talking. Have enough light so that they can see your face, and do not cover your mouth when speaking. Avoid talking to the person from another room.
- Remove yourself to a quiet area to reduce the distraction of background noise. In a social situation, a one-to-one conversation away from the noise of the group may be easier than a group conversation.
- Keep your information short and simple, and allow pauses between pieces of information for the listener to process what is heard.
- Avoid shouting, as this can distort the sounds further, and confuse the listener. Raise your voice a little and speak more slowly.
- Check that the person has heard you and understood. Ask the listener for feedback: 'Does that make sense?' or 'Was I clear in what I said?'
- Have hearing assessed regularly, as hearing acuity can change, especially with age or illness.
- If hearing aids have been recommended, ensure they are working properly and are being worn.

It is worth checking any **medications** that are being taken for their possible **side-effects** on memory. Valium (diazepam) is a commonly used drug that can have a negative effect on remembering.[11]

Lifestyle (unfamiliar environment)

Gordon's memory started to get worse at about the same time as he and his wife moved into their new unit. Being in a new or unfamiliar environment can make remembering more difficult, especially for people who have had a brain injury, such as a stroke. When you move house, there is so much that is new to you. Learning where everything is kept can be a major undertaking, particularly when you have lived in your previous house for a very long time. People with memory difficulties can experience a similar sense of stress on their memory with any change of routine or new environment, such as moving home, going away on holiday or being admitted to hospital.

Attitude

Lilian has noticed that Gordon is not wanting to work on improving his situation, but rather blames all his problems on his stroke, and says, 'There's nothing I can do about it.' While he holds a non-motivated attitude, he will probably not actively seek out any advice. It may be that Lilian will have to be the one who instigates change.

Lilian will benefit from discussing her feelings and attitudes towards Gordon with an experienced counsellor. This could help her to understand the changes she has noticed in Gordon. She may not have realised the extra load that moving house was going to place on Gordon's memory, or the possible effect of his feelings of grief and loss on his motivation levels. She could work with the counsellor on introducing practical memory strategies to support the changes she has observed in Gordon's everyday memory ability.

For example, she could set up a written reminder system on a wall calendar, so that she can reinforce what she tells Gordon by having it written down for him as well. She might also like to put labels in the cupboards and other storage areas to help Gordon get to know where items are stored in the new unit.

Lilian could also encourage Gordon to:

- see his doctor to check if any medical complications are making his memory worse, including possible grief and mood issues
- ask his doctor about possible side-effects of Valium (diazepam) on his memory
- arrange to have his hearing checked, to see if he would benefit from a hearing aid
- take part in regular activities, such as attending the local 'Men's Shed' group, or joining the bowls or golf club with friends.

See Chapters 6 and 9 for further information about supporting someone who has memory loss.

Possible reasons for memory change

The stories in this chapter have highlighted several reasons why our memory may not always function at its best. Take the time now to run through the following checklist, and mentally note any factors that might be having an adverse effect on your memory at the moment.

- Are you unwell?
- Are you taking any medication and, if so, do you know if it can affect your memory?
- Do you drink too much alcohol, or use other drugs to excess?
- Is your hearing or vision impaired in any way?
- Do you have pain?
- Are you eating and exercising well?
- Could your hormone levels be altered at the moment?
- Do you think you might be depressed, or do you often feel 'down in the dumps'?
- Are you experiencing a high level of anxiety, fear or distress?
- Is your sleep disturbed?

- Is your workload too heavy?
- Is your current level of mental stimulation adequate for you?
- Do you have low expectations about how your memory will work for you?

To get the most out of your memory, you might need to take action. You may need to change your thoughts about yourself and your memory. Having realistic rather than negative expectations about memory functioning can help you be more relaxed about it. A change in what you think and what you say to yourself can actually enhance your memory.

Many factors can reduce your capacity to attend to what is going on around you. It may be this reduction in attention that is having an effect on your memory at the moment. You may need to find ways to increase your attention to what you want to get into your memory storage.

If you think your workload could explain why your memory is not at its best, then consider ways to reduce it. Think about time management, pace yourself, and include brief times to relax properly, at your desk, in the car park, at the bus stop. Being relaxed has a positive effect on your attention level. You might like to investigate some specific relaxation techniques, such as deep-muscle relaxation, meditation, mindfulness, breathing practices or yoga.

During times when you feel your memory is letting you down, be kind to yourself, and introduce supportive memory strategies. Chapter 6 describes specific strategies to help nurture your memory. A visit to your doctor will help establish whether there are any health issues that could be affecting your memory. Of course there are sometimes factors that are beyond our control, but there are often things that you can do with your health, lifestyle and attitude towards remembering that can help you get more out of your memory.

Key points   WHAT ELSE AFFECTS MEMORY?

- At any age, our ability to remember can fluctuate.
- Our memory abilities are influenced by various factors, some of which are under our own control—including aspects of our health, our lifestyle and, importantly, our attitudes and beliefs in our own skills.
- To get the most out of your memory, it is important to be aware of these factors and, if necessary, actively do something about them.

CHAPTER 4

Memory during menopause

My life is out of control because of my forgetting.
Donna, 44

Mum, have you got Alzheimer's or something? I've told you that already, don't you remember?
Charlotte, 17

I've never been able to talk to anyone about this, and no one told me what to expect. I've been scared that I'm going around the bend.
Clara, 54

Some people just breeze through menopause—maybe that's why women don't talk to each other about it, because we don't all have the same experience.
Anjali, 59

There is so much stigma—it's like menopause is a dirty word. I am surrounded by younger people at work; I try to hide my memory failures. There is no way I would talk to people at work about menopause—they probably wouldn't know what it means.
Abuya, 48

What is menopause?

We learn about the changes that happen to us at puberty when we are at school, but most of us haven't been taught about menopause. What do you know about menopause? Have a go at this short quiz to check your knowledge! Choose true or false for the following 10 questions. The answers are provided over the page.

1 Menopause marks the end of a woman's reproductive years. *True or False?*

2 The average age of menopause (defined as 12 consecutive months without a menstrual period) is 59. *True or False?*

3 During the time leading up to menopause, the levels of hormones produced by the ovaries fluctuate. *True or False?*

4 'Perimenopause'—the transition phase close to menopause, when menstrual patterns typically become irregular (in the length of the period, the time between periods, and the level of flow)—always lasts for five years. *True or False?*

5 'Premenopause' is the time before perimenopause. *True or False?*

6 After menopause, women are said to be 'postmenopausal'. *True or False?*

7 Women can experience premature or early menopause after surgical removal of the ovaries, or chemotherapy or radio-therapy treatment for cancer. *True or False?*

8 All women experience hot flushes during menopause. *True or False?*

9 Mood changes, irritability and anxiety are not common during menopause. *True or False?*

10 Many women complain of forgetfulness during menopause. *True or False?*

This chapter will answer questions such as:

- How many women notice forgetfulness during menopause?
- How do women feel about their memory during menopause?
- What type of memory difficulties do women notice at midlife?
- Is there any evidence that memory is worse during menopause?
- What helps when you notice forgetfulness around menopause?

Research on memory during menopause

Over the past few decades, researchers have begun to study memory during menopause in more detail, and in recent years I have conducted research on this topic. It all started with my involvement in education sessions for women about memory and menopause at the Royal Women's Hospital in Melbourne, Australia. These sessions were part of a broader education program about menopause, covering practical information and tips for a range of menopause symptoms. For several years, I provided these sessions together with Associate Professor Christina Bryant, a friend and colleague who is a clinical psychologist. Our topic was 'Mood and memory during menopause'. We found that the women attending the sessions benefited from gaining a better understanding of what can happen in terms of mood and memory, and what is helpful when you experience these symptoms. As Christina continued her work in the Menopause Clinic at the hospital, she noticed that women coming to see her would describe forgetfulness and concern about memory. Being an academic as well as a clinician, Christina suggested that I do some research on this topic. So I spent several years doing just that, completing my PhD in 2013 on memory during menopause.

My doctorate research project was conducted at the hospital, and I saw 130 women, who attended either menopause or gynaecology clinics.[1] The women ranged in age from 40 to 60, and were divided into groups according to their stage of menopause. There were 36 premenopausal, 54 perimenopausal and 40 postmenopausal

Answers

1 *Menopause marks the end of a woman's reproductive years.*
   True. The first menstrual period during puberty marks the start
   of a woman's reproductive years, and the last menstrual period
   signifies the end of the reproductive years.

2 *The average age of menopause (defined as 12 consecutive months
   without a menstrual period) is 59.*
   False. The average age for a woman to reach menopause is
   around 50, but the most common age range for menopause
   to occur is between 48 and 55.

3 *During the time leading up to menopause, the levels of hormones
   produced by the ovaries fluctuate.*
   True. Levels of hormones, including oestrogen and progesterone,
   fluctuate during the time leading up to menopause. The overall
   levels of these hormones decrease during the menopausal transition and, after menopause, oestrogen and progesterone are no
   longer produced by the ovaries.

4 *'Perimenopause'—the transition phase close to menopause, when
   menstrual patterns typically become irregular (in the length of the
   period, the time between periods, and the level of flow)—always
   lasts for five years.*
   False. This transition stage varies in length and can last for up
   to 10 years.

5 *'Premenopause' is the time before perimenopause.*
   True. Premenopause is the stage of women's reproductive years
   that begins with the first menstrual cycle and ends around the
   time that perimenopause begins.

6 *After menopause, women are said to be 'postmenopausal'.*
   True. A woman is considered to be postmenopausal after she
   has reached menopause, which is defined by looking back and

knowing that there have been 12 consecutive months without a menstrual period.

7 *Women can experience premature or early menopause after surgical removal of the ovaries, or chemotherapy or radiotherapy treatment for cancer.*
True. These medical procedures can lead to menopause. Before the age of 40, it is called 'premature menopause', and before the age of 45, it is called 'early menopause'.

8 *All women experience hot flushes during menopause.*
False. Hot flushes, giving a sudden warm feeling, are not experienced by all women during menopause. They are very common though, and about 85 per cent of women report having hot flushes and night-time sweats. Sleeping difficulties are also common around menopause.

9 *Mood changes, irritability and anxiety are not common during menopause.*
False. A combination of hormonal changes and sleep deprivation can contribute to mood changes, irritability and anxiety around the time of menopause. These problems can become worse at times of stress, and it is common to experience stress during this life stage. Life is full, with work both inside and outside the home, and family commitments, including children and older parents.

10 *Many women complain of forgetfulness during menopause.*
True. Many women notice forgetfulness around the time of menopause, and that's what this chapter is about! It's common to wonder whether memory lapses are part of menopause. Some women start to fear that their forgetfulness may be an early sign of dementia.

women. Each woman completed questionnaires focusing on their feelings about memory, and underwent a detailed neuropsychological assessment of their memory abilities.

How many women notice forgetfulness during menopause?

The responses given by the sample of women from the Royal Women's Hospital helped to answer several questions about memory during menopause. First, we looked at the proportion of women who acknowledged that they had experienced 'poor memory in the past month'. Combining the responses of all women, including those who were premenopausal, perimenopausal and postmenopausal, about three-quarters of women (72 per cent to be exact) said they had experienced poor memory in the past month. So, a clear majority of women in this study had recently noticed poor memory.

Here is the breakdown of each group.

Have you experienced poor memory in the past month?	Yes
Premenopausal group	62%
Perimenopausal group	82%
Postmenopausal group	68%

You can see that it was women in the perimenopausal stage who reported the highest memory complaints, at 82 per cent. You might expect that the women in this clinic sample would complain more about memory than women in the general community, since they had come to a hospital clinic and may have been experiencing more intense menopause symptoms. When we looked at other studies, we found that the proportion of perimenopausal women reporting memory symptoms in this study was similar to, or slightly higher than, that observed in other Australian and US community-based studies.[2] So, the answer to the question, 'How many women notice forgetfulness during menopause?', would have to be 'most'—and especially women who are in the peri-menopausal transition stage.

How do women feel about their memory during menopause?

In our study at the Royal Women's Hospital, we looked at how satisfied women were with their memory using a detailed questionnaire about beliefs and confidence in memory. We found that perimenopausal women were significantly less satisfied with their memory than premenopausal and postmenopausal women. When we looked at general community responses on this same questionnaire,[3] we noticed that memory satisfaction in the perimenopausal women in our study was well below that in the community, indicating significant memory dissatisfaction for these women.

Women in the study had to rate the degree to which they agreed with 18 statements tapping into their beliefs and feelings about memory. The statements the perimenopausal women agreed to most strongly indicated they felt that their memory was not working as well as it used to. They acknowledged feeling unhappy, concerned, embarrassed, and lacking in confidence in relation to their memory ability. They agreed that they had hidden their memory problems so others wouldn't notice.

I'll be driving to a place that I've been to lots of times. I start to go there and then suddenly I can't remember what direction it is in. You think you're going nuts.
Pia, 52

I feel like there is a hole in my head. I think I need to have a brain scan to check. I feel like I'm losing my mind and I have Alzheimer's. I get really upset when I forget things at work. It makes me feel insecure and sad.
June, 46

I write a shopping list and think I must put it in my purse. When I get to the shops I see that it's not in my purse and realise that I have forgotten to put it in my purse. It worries me that I didn't remember that I forgot to do this.

Fiona, 49

I can't even call my kids the right name. The wrong words are coming out. I'm calling Bradley Phil. I go blank on people's names—I'm so embarrassed. I know I just can't get them, can't access them. Sometimes I don't even pick it up straight away.

Anya, 48

I'm conscious not to say the wrong thing at work. I'm hesitant. I don't want them to hear me say the wrong thing.

Jo, 52

What type of memory difficulties do women notice at midlife?

We asked all of the women in our study to rate how frequently they experienced 20 everyday memory lapses. We found that not only did the perimenopausal women report less satisfaction with their memory, they also reported significantly more frequent memory lapses than the premenopausal and postmenopausal women. Women in the premenopausal and postmenopausal groups reported a similar frequency of memory lapses to people in the general community, but the perimenopausal women in our study reported more frequent memory difficulties than people in the general community.[4]

The most frequently acknowledged memory lapses by the perimenopausal women included:

- trouble recalling names and specific words
- forgetting what they were just about to do, like walking into a room and forgetting what they went in there for
- forgetting a phone number they had just looked up

- leaving something behind they meant to take with them
- forgetting something they read earlier in the day, or something they intended to buy
- trouble concentrating
- losing their train of thought
- forgetting what they were about to say.

Now—you can tell me a name and I forget it in seconds!
Tamar, 50

I will have a blank for the word I want to say and it just won't come.
Lena, 55

I go upstairs and I think, 'What did I come up here for?'
Debbie, 44

It's just like it sits there and doesn't sink in. It took me three months to learn my mobile phone number.
Angela, 51

I keep forgetting to take things with me—like when we go to our holiday house, I forget to take the phone charger.
Siobhan, 48

I used to have a photographic memory, and now I read a novel and can't recall what I was reading.
Vicki, 54

I forget things. My son asked me to get some ham at the supermarket and I got half a dozen things, but when I got home I realised I had forgotten to get the ham. I forget to do things even though I've said I will do them. Some of this is because I'm really busy.
May Lin, 50

I forget what I'm talking about mid-sentence and totally lose my train of thought.
Tracey, 50

If I get symptoms of menopause, like a hot flush, I get anxious and worry about what I appear like in front of people and then I don't concentrate. Have they noticed that my hair is dripping? Have I turned red? And do they know that my heart is pumping?

Anuja, 52

Is there evidence that memory function is worse during menopause?

We know that many women notice forgetfulness during the menopausal transition. We also know that there is a decrease in hormones, such as oestrogen, as women experience menopause, and these hormones are important for optimal brain functioning, especially in regions of the brain that are known to be important to memory. Researchers have suggested that these alterations in oestrogen levels could be detrimental to memory ability.[5]

So is there any evidence that memory becomes worse during menopause? There have been relatively few studies that have directly investigated this question, and the studies that have been performed have reported conflicting findings. Some cross-sectional studies have compared groups of women who are in different stages of menopause. Other longitudinal studies have observed the same group of women as they move through the natural stages of menopause. Each study has tested memory in a different way, which makes it difficult to compare one study to another, and to draw firm conclusions.

In our study at the Royal Women's Hospital, we gave 130 women a challenging and detailed set of memory tests that took 90 minutes to complete. We included tests that covered the types of memory processes involved in the various everyday memory lapses that women tend to report. The women completed tasks that measured attention and concentration, speed of processing information, planning and organisational skills, and the ability to learn new information, to remember to do something at a specific time, to find specific words when put on the spot, to switch from one way of doing something to another, and to remember something when you haven't been told to try to remember it for later.

We found no difference in performance between the premenopausal, perimenopausal and postmenopausal groups on any of these memory tests. This finding was similar to several other studies that have found no evidence of worsening memory during the menopausal transition. This is reassuring, but it doesn't rule out the possibility that some women may experience subtle change in some aspects of memory. Indeed, some studies in which the same memory tests have been given to individual women as they transitioned through menopause have reported very small changes in women's memory during perimenopause and early postmenopause.[6]

Why do women feel less confident about their memory during menopause?

Menopause is a time of transition. It's a time when many women become aware of changes in themselves. Physical symptoms of menopause, such as changes in menstrual cycles and hot flushes, can be seen as the first signs of ageing. When women focus on these signs of getting older, perhaps they start to focus more on other aspects of their life, like memory lapses. Studies looking at perceptions of memory have shown that both men and women can become concerned about their memory at midlife,[7] and the often negative stereotypes of ageing in some societies only serve to make people feel worse about their memory.

It's not just feeling negative about getting older that may affect our perceptions about memory. In our study, we found that a woman's attitude towards menopause was an additional factor that related to feelings about memory. Women in the perimenopausal group who reported a more positive attitude towards menopause tended to say that they felt more confident and positive about their memory, when compared to women who reported a more negative attitude towards menopause.

The perimenopausal women in our study who performed most poorly on a measure of attention were the women who tended to report more forgetfulness. Memory lapses are often related to not paying enough attention, and there are many reasons why women find it difficult to pay attention during menopause. Our study showed that perimenopausal women who reported more anxiety and mood symptoms, and more sleep disturbance and hot flushes, reported more negative feelings about their memory. Of course, anxiety, depression and poor sleep can make it difficult to pay attention and focus. Add to that the demanding lives women often lead at midlife, working both in and out of the home, and being there for children, parents and friends, and we can see why midlife memory lapses related to not paying full attention can occur!

Our research also showed that women going through menopause reported less control over their memory than women who had not yet reached the menopausal transition.

At times I get anxious and frustrated because I feel that I am unable to control aspects of my life anymore, like vagueness, loss of concentration, and at times memory lapses for things like names.
Libby, 47

The more I noticed my memory problem, the more I got anxious.
Bea, 55

I'm scared about having Alzheimer's.
Bernadetta, 58

Concern and anxiety about memory during menopause can have a real impact on self-confidence. When your confidence is low, it can affect your work performance, personal relationships and everyday functioning. In a large study in the United Kingdom, 40 per cent of the perimenopausal and postmenopausal women who took part reported a negative impact of menopause on their work perform-ance, which was particularly related to perceived difficulties with concentration and memory.[8]

I left my job because of these changes. I couldn't do what I was in charge of doing—it was so overwhelming. There were hundreds of women at my work and they wouldn't talk about menopause or losing memory. I got no support from my work. They wouldn't admit to it being something we all go through.
Cynthia, 58

What helps when you notice forgetfulness around menopause?

I don't just want their sympathy—I want to know why it's happening and is there anything I can do to make it better.
Melinda, 54

The results of my doctorate research project pointed to a clear need to support women regarding memory concerns during the meno-pausal transition. Fortunately, I had been involved in conducting memory support groups for older adults for several years, using a program devised by a Melbourne-based group of researchers.[9] After consulting this research team, we decided to trial the memory support group at the Royal Women's Hospital with groups of women who were experiencing menopause. Women attended the group once a week for four weeks. We discussed how memory works, normal age-related changes in memory, and memory illnesses, such as dementia. The women were trained to use a range of specific memory strategies, and provided with information about enhan-cing memory by focusing on health and lifestyle factors. The results were clear: attending the memory support group improved the women's beliefs and self-confidence around memory.[10]

What I've learned from coming to this course:

- Not to be so hard on myself, the importance of mindfulness, and knowing when my memory is more likely to let me down.
- I have always prided myself in my memory. It has always been a strength. You have taught me that some aspects of the change in my memory are natural and I have no control over them, but I don't feel so much like I'm on the edge of a cliff because you have shown me there are many aspects I can control.

Tanya, 49

So, what did we do in the groups to bring about this change in women's self-confidence around memory? What helps when you're concerned about memory during menopause?

Understand your memory

Talk about memory with other women who are going through menopause. Women attending the memory groups found it reassuring to know that other women had similar memory lapses and shared their concern about memory.

I feel better knowing that others have the same issues with memory. I have been telling all my friends what we are doing in the sessions, and helping them to understand about memory, too.

Jocelyn, 55

Learn how memory works (outlined in Chapter 1 of this book). It is normal for memory to fluctuate, especially if you are having difficulty paying attention. Forgetting is a normal part of the memory system that prevents overload.

Now I know that it is normal to have a few memory lapses.

Hoa, 50

This is really good timing—I wouldn't have wanted to know this when I was 30, but now it's good information for me, for my parents and for my children.
Vivian, 50

Learn about the difference between everyday memory lapses that can be age-related (see Chapter 2) and more significant memory loss, which can occur with dementia and other memory illnesses (see Chapter 8).

I feel so relieved to know that my memory lapses are normal.
Mandy, 49

Develop more realistic expectations of your memory. Our research on memory during menopause showed that women with higher expectations of their memory tended to feel worse about their memory. You may feel better about your memory if you don't put so much pressure on yourself.

Celia, aged 52, had worked in childcare for most of her career and had started to worry about her memory because she was finding it hard to recall over 100 children's names, and the names of the children's parents. She had always prided herself in her memory for names. After learning about how memory works and normal age-related changes in encoding and retrieval, Celia said that she felt reassured about her memory. She felt that it was okay not to be able to learn all those names in a short period of time.
Anne

Pay attention to paying attention!

When we remember something new, we need to pay attention to it. For example, when people introduce themselves to you, you need to pay attention to their name and their face. If anything stops you from paying full attention, then you will be less likely to remember their name later on because you never got the name into memory storage in the first place.

I was so nervous about how the meeting would go that when people came into the room and started introducing themselves to me, I wasn't able to focus on what they were saying.
Lin, 44

Of course, life gets in the way, and we are not always able to pay attention and focus. Many midlife memory lapses are related to not paying full attention. It helps if you make a conscious effort to pay attention.

I was at a social gathering during the week and was introduced to a woman. I told her that I am doing a memory course and I have been told to make associations with names. She told me her name was Sherry and I told her I would remember her name because I like drinking Sherry! We laughed and she told me that she has trouble remembering names, too.
Peggy, 51

Feeling anxious about your memory can set up a cycle, where your memory can start to let you down even more. Your anxiety about remembering can prevent you from being able to pay full attention to incoming information, which in itself can lead to memory lapses. When you experience another memory lapse, this gives you more evidence that your memory is a problem, and then you feel even more anxious about your memory.

It's a vicious circle—I feel self-doubt and self-consciousness. I run myself down and then I forget something again. I'll be in a conversation or a meeting, and I think, 'I need to remember this'. I become so anxious that I'm not going to remember it and I stop listening and shut it out and later I don't remember.

Samantha, 55

To help interrupt this 'memory–anxiety spiral', take the time to pay full attention and learn something new. You could try learning a mobile phone number or the name of someone who is important to you. Take your time to do this, and show yourself that your memory can work. See Chapter 6 for strategies to assist with achieving this new learning.

Robyn's 16-year-old daughter, Ava, criticised her repeatedly about not remembering what she had said to her. Robyn decided to show Ava that she could remember. Next time Ava spoke to her, Robyn stopped doing what she was doing and made an effort to focus her full attention on what her daughter was saying.

Anne

At a dinner, I met a woman with an unusual name. She said, 'You won't remember my name.' I replied, 'Yes I will.' I focused on it, said it a few times and remembered to say goodbye to her. She was impressed. I felt good.

Kiara, 51

Use memory strategies

At midlife, many women use strategies to support their memory. In our research study at the Royal Women's Hospital, the peri-menopausal women reported that their most frequently used memory strategy was a written reminder. Women reported using reminders in calendars, diaries, notebooks and shopping lists. These 'external' memory strategies, that involve using some sort of external aid to help memory, are the most commonly used techniques to support everyday memory. Other external strategies involve putting something in a special place as a reminder to do something, using technical reminder systems, and asking someone to remind you.

Tamara, aged 57, came to the memory group saying that she didn't want to have to rely on writing information down. She had started a new job, working on reception, and had to learn several new procedures. She was trying to keep all the new information in her head, but found that she kept getting distracted by phone calls and customers arriving at her desk. After some encouragement to try external memory strategies, Tamara organised her work systems and compiled a written procedure manual. She told the group how positive this process had been. She now felt more confident, and said that her mind was freed up for work.

Anne

Lily, aged 50, said she has always had a good memory and has never used written reminders. When her mother became seriously ill, Lily started to feel overwhelmed. When she went to bed each night, she would run through all the things she had to do in her mind, but she kept feeling she would forget something important, like to take her mother to a medical appointment. After taking up on the suggestion to use an organised written reminder app in her mobile phone, Lily expressed relief, saying, 'It's so good to dump the information from my head somewhere else, and to stop going over and over it when I lie in bed at night.'

Anne

I've got a work conference coming up next week that I'm on the organising committee for, so I know that I'm going to need to use all my reminder systems more because I'll be overloaded.

Connie, 59

Most women use a combination of 'external' and 'internal' memory strategies to assist memory. Internal strategies come from within us. They often involve adding meaning to information using visualisation and association. These strategies help by focusing our attention to information, and processing the information more deeply. For example, to remember where you parked your car in section 'E2' of a multi-storey car park, you might visualise two elephants sitting on your car! Chapter 6 provides more information about memory strategies.

Megan, aged 47, was having difficulty recalling the name of the man who always served her when she went to the motorbike parts shop. His name is James. We came up with the idea of imagining he is 'James Dean' the actor, riding on his motorbike, and she said she no longer has any trouble remembering his name!
Anne

Midlife memory also benefits from a supportive environment, both at home and at work. We can design our environment and the appliances that we use to reduce the load on our memory. For example, at work it helps to have a list of all staff displayed, with their photos next to their names to help us remember our colleague's names. At home, we don't have to remember to turn the iron off, if we use an iron that turns itself off when we forget! See Chapters 7 and 10 for more information about memory strategies at work and memory-wise environments.

Run through the midlife memory-health checklist!

We all notice fluctuations in our ability to remember from time to time, and especially at midlife. Our memory abilities can be less efficient when we are excessively busy, emotionally stressed, or mentally or physically unwell. In particular, it can be difficult to pay attention and focus at these times. It's common to feel a sense of loss during the menopausal transition. Your role as a parent is changing as your children become more independent, and you may be reassessing your work role or planning your retirement. You might be stressed and busy with supporting your parents and feeling negative about going through menopause and getting older. Our memory processes are sensitive to what is happening in our lives and to our physical and emotional wellbeing.

Take a moment to run through this midlife memory health check:

- Is your workload too heavy?
- Are you experiencing a high level of stress or anxiety?
- Is your sleep disturbed?
- Are you feeling constantly sad or depressed?
- Are you unwell?
- Do you have pain?
- Is your vision or hearing impaired in any way?
- Are you taking any medication and, if so, do you know if it can affect your memory?
- Do you drink too much alcohol, or use other drugs to excess?

If you are concerned about your memory and you answered yes to any of these questions, it might be time to take action. The previous chapter provides more information about factors such as anxiety, depression, sleep, stress, alcohol, pain and medications. Of course there are sometimes aspects of our lives that are beyond our control, but there are often things that we can do with our health, lifestyle and emotional balance that can help us get more out of our memory. Be proactive and work on the things that you can control!

When you're not feeling right, you don't think right.
Ruth, 56

My memory got worse in my fifties, and I put it down to menopause. My hearing has been a slight problem for many years, and when I learned that hearing is important for memory during the memory group, I decided to get my hearing tested. I had been finding it hard to hear on the phone, and I didn't realise how bad my hearing was until the audiologist put some hearing aids on me and I could hear! The audiologist explained how my hearing loss could affect my memory and I got quite emotional.

I felt so relieved to know what had caused my memory problem, and that I could now finally do something about it.
Camilla, 56

Before hormone replacement therapy (HRT), I had terrible sleep. I woke up every hour with hot flushes and was so sleep deprived. I found it harder to remember things I should do. This has improved with HRT, and getting better sleep. It was definitely sleep-related.
Kaye, 55

My memory is okay now. When I started being menopausal, I was concerned. You have to realise that if there's something wrong with your health or if you are overloaded, it will affect your memory. Self-preservation is important—be kind to yourself.
Maia, 59

Nurture your brain health at midlife and beyond!

After taking the time to think about your memory during menopause, to work on strategies to support your memory, and to make adjustments to aspects of your health and lifestyle that may lead to improved memory, you might just find yourself feeling better about your memory than you did before. The challenge now is to maintain this feeling as you get older.

I've been doing all these things because of coming to this group. It has spurred me on to get organised. I feel so much more organised and motivated for the future.
Sheryl, 51

You can read more about nurturing brain health in Chapter 5, but for now, let's focus on the key evidence-based strategies that have been proposed for maintaining your memory and reducing your chances of developing dementia.

- The healthier your body is, the healthier your brain will be. Around midlife, there can be changes in your blood pressure, blood glucose and cholesterol levels, so see your doctor regularly to manage these aspects of your health. Exercise regularly, enjoy a healthy diet, avoid smoking and keep alcohol intake low.
- Your psychological wellbeing is important for your brain health. Seek treatment for persisting stress, anxiety or depressive symptoms.
- Stay connected socially and take part in regular activities that involve new experiences and mental effort.

Further support and information

See your doctor if you remain concerned about your memory, or if you would like further information about menopause, anxiety, depression, hot flushes or sleep disturbance.

Your local women's health or menopause support organisation and your local dementia support organisation can provide further information and support. Details of such support organisations are provided in the 'Resources' section at the end of this book.

Key points   MEMORY DURING MENOPAUSE

- It is common to notice forgetfulness during menopause.
- Around menopause, many women feel concerned, embarrassed and lacking in confidence about memory.
- Common memory lapses reported by women at midlife include difficulty recalling names, specific words, what you were just about to do, what you were meant to buy or take with you, something you read recently, trouble concentrating, losing your train of thought and forgetting what you were about to say.

- Studies that have examined memory during menopause by asking women to complete memory tests have reported conflicting findings. Many studies have found no evidence of poor memory performance during menopause, but some studies have reported subtle changes in some aspects of memory.
- Self-confidence about memory at midlife can be enhanced by:
  - learning more about how memory works, and developing realistic expectations of your memory
  - paying attention to paying attention!
  - using a variety of specific memory strategies to support your memory
  - identifying and managing any aspects of your health and lifestyle that could be impacting on your memory.
- Midlife is an opportune time to take positive steps for your future brain health.

CHAPTER 5

What can we do to reduce the risk of developing dementia?

In Chapters 3 and 4, the focus was on how to get the most out of your memory as you are right now. In this chapter, the emphasis will be on your future memory and brain health, answering questions such as, 'What can I do to minimise the impact of ageing on my memory?' and, 'Is there anything I can do to reduce my risk of developing dementia?'

In my clinical practice as a neuropsychologist I see people who are concerned about their memory. Some people have no detectable memory difficulties, others have mild inefficiency related to a variety of issues, and others have significant memory loss associated with memory illnesses, like dementia. When I ask people what they want to get out of the neuropsychological consultation, most will say, 'I want to know what I can do to stop my memory from getting worse.'

Most of us don't ask ourselves this question until we reach midlife, and experience a few memory lapses, or perhaps a friend or family member is diagnosed with dementia. We might start to have a few health issues and think more about our future health, including our brain health. Brain and memory function are sensitive to how we live our life and to other aspects of our physical and mental health. The earlier you begin to work on optimising your brain health, the better. Midlife is an opportune time because this is often when changes in our health occur that can begin to have a negative impact on the brain.

Risk factors for Alzheimer's disease

While research into medical treatment for dementia continues, there is currently no drug available to prevent or cure Alzheimer's disease. Some risks for dementia are genetic and are not currently modifiable. Whether you end up developing a brain disease like dementia comes down to a combination of your genes and other non-genetic factors. Decades of international dementia research studies suggest that there is the potential to modify negative non-genetic influences in order to reduce your chance of developing dementia, or at least delay the onset of the disease.[1]

Scientists examining these potential non-genetic influences have discovered relationships between particular health and lifestyle risk factors, the brain disease process, and subsequent development of dementia. Around one-third of all dementia cases are associated with a combination of these risk factors.[2] Researchers suggest it is best to address as many of these risk factors as possible, aiming to enhance brain health and reduce the risk of developing dementia or delay its onset.[3] We will discuss these specific risk factors in more detail later in the chapter.

The latest research into reducing dementia risk has focused on ways that we can build up 'brain resilience' in an effort to prevent or delay the onset of symptoms. When people have dementia, the changes that occur in the brain build up over a long period of time. Typically, people start showing symptoms of the illness, such as memory loss, decades after these changes begin.[4] If we work on building up our 'brain resilience', then we may lessen the impact of disease processes on everyday functioning. If we can harness the brain's ability to form new connections between nerve networks, then perhaps we can build up resilience to dementia. The methods for building up brain resilience identified by research will be covered later in this chapter.

While it feels good to be proactive and to work on a healthy ageing plan, it's important to acknowledge that none of us have total control over our future health. We all know someone who has done all the 'right' things, but still develops an illness such as dementia. This person may have followed all the evidence-based suggestions for maintaining brain health, but ended up having dementia. It's the same with other illnesses. We know so much now about reducing our risk for heart attack, for example, but it is not really possible to prevent a heart attack with certainty.[5]

Ultimately, there is a limit to the extent we can control our health. Addressing the health and lifestyle risk factors for dementia identified by research might only have the potential to delay or reduce the change of developing dementia in one-third of all cases of the disease.[6] The condition is very complex, and we do not fully understand how it develops. It's important not to blame yourself if you have dementia, and similarly important not to think that others who have dementia have brought it on themselves. Sometimes our genes win out against all the other non-genetic factors that we diligently work on.

We may not be able to stop ourselves from getting an illness like Alzheimer's disease, and much more research needs to be done to help us understand more clearly what we can do to prevent dementia. In the meantime, we can do what the current research suggests, and hope that we may be able to delay the onset of the symptoms of dementia, so that even if we have the illness in the brain, it has less impact on our lives, and the lives of those closest to us.

Your personalised future brain health plan

Your memory and brain health are like any other aspect of your health: they can change with age. We all change as we get older. We can't stop the ageing process totally—but we can be proactive about brain health. We can have regular check-ups and perform necessary adjustments to keep our brain as healthy as possible, just like we take our car to the mechanic for regular maintenance and care. We have routine health checks for various parts of our bodies as we get older, and it helps if we include memory and brain maintenance on our list of parts that need to be taken care of!

You've probably read those lists of tips for memory health in articles about ageing and dementia. These provide a helpful general guide for everyone. But you are not everyone—you are *you*! A strategy that suits one person may not suit another. To keep your brain as healthy as possible, and to work on the suggested methods for reducing the chance of memory illnesses, such as dementia, you need a personalised plan of attack! The best first step for this is to book a long appointment with your doctor.

Health factors found to be associated with risk of developing dementia include high blood pressure, high cholesterol, diabetes, obesity, smoking, excessive alcohol consumption, depression, anxiety and stress.[7] Some of these factors can cause changes in your brain. If that occurs, you might not get optimum function from it as you get older and you could have less resilience to brain illnesses, such as dementia. It is important to identify these factors, so you can start to work on reducing any possible effect that they may have on your future brain health and your health in general.

Your doctor will check through your personal and medical history with you, and ask you questions about your normal daily and weekly routine. This check-up usually involves a physical examination. You might even end up doing some memory tests. You may be asked to have further medical investigations done to complete the information gathering stage. Your doctor might not have time to complete a comprehensive check-up, and you may be referred to a medical specialist who works in the field of ageing and dementia.

Based on the information you and your doctors compile, you can work together on a plan to modify any features of your health and lifestyle that can be altered, which will aim to enhance your brain health and boost your 'brain resilience' for the future. The research on brain health shows that individuals have the most success in working towards these goals when the plan is specific for them, and this customised approach targets several aspects of their health and lifestyle at once.[8] Once you know the areas you need to work on, it may help if you see specialists in those fields to assist with making the recommended changes. For example, a psychiatrist or psychologist can assist with managing stress, or symptoms of depression and anxiety.

Building up 'brain resilience'

The next step is to consider what you can do in an effort to build up your brain's resilience to disease. Scientists have proposed that we may be able to prevent or delay the onset of the symptoms of dementia, if we can build up 'brain resilience'. The idea here is that a person may have changes in their brain that indicate dementia, such as Alzheimer's disease, but the actual symptoms of the dementia developing, such as memory loss, may emerge later if a person has built up sufficient resilience to the disease over their lifetime.[9]

Let's run through the aspects of daily life that numerous studies have shown to be important for building up such 'brain resilience'. And remember, the research tells us that it is best to work on as many of these areas as possible, not to just focus on one or two.

Physical exercise
Regular physical exercise can boost general cardiovascular fitness, and in turn increase blood flow to the brain. Studies have suggested

that exercise can increase levels of a protein in the brain called the 'brain-derived neurotrophic factor'.[10] This protein promotes growth and survival of brain cells and may strengthen the brain's resilience to injury or disease.

Increasing the amount of physical exercise you do from midlife onwards is associated with a reduced risk of dementia, possibly because it can have a positive impact on some of the health issues associated with increased risk for dementia, such as obesity, insulin resistance, high blood pressure and high cholesterol.[11]

When it comes to maximising everyday memory performance in healthy older adults or people with dementia, there is still no clear consensus about the possible effect of physical exercise. Some studies describe improved performance on memory tests after older adults have taken part in several months of regular aerobic exercise, whereas others report that exercise alone does not improve memory performance. Nevertheless, regular physical exercise enhances general fitness and mood.[12]

Talk to your doctor about the best way for you to include daily exercise in your routine. Scientists have suggested that we include a combination of aerobic, strength and balance exercises.[13] Exercising under the guidance of a physiotherapist or exercise physiologist will ensure that you do this safely, and in a way that suits your body and your routine.

Mental stimulation

Mental stimulation can come from a variety of activities, including taking part in new and varied pastimes, education courses, and attending programs that provide training on specific memory and thinking tasks. Mental stimulation over a lifetime has been associated with promoting resilience to brain illnesses, such as dementia, and delaying the onset of symptoms of the illness.[14] These findings suggest that 'brain resilience' to dementia is something that continues to build up over your lifetime, from the years that you spent at school completing formal education, to the new learning activities that you do now to stimulate your brain.

Scientists have shown that when we challenge ourselves for months or years with new experiences that involve mental effort, changes occur in the brain to support the learning of the new skill.[15] These changes can involve increases in the number of brain cells and supporting cells, and stronger connections between the brain cells. This type of brain plasticity is possible throughout life, and the brain changes that occur with prolonged mental activity could build up resilience to disease processes that cause dementia.

We are spoilt for choice when it comes to mentally stimulating activities that could build up 'brain resilience'. We can read a challenging book, complete regular brain-teaser puzzles, or do mentally engaging cooking or craft activities. We can enrol in educational courses, or perhaps learn a new language or musical instrument. Volunteer work usually involves learning something new, as does travelling to somewhere you haven't been before. It's important to choose activities that work for you. If the challenge is too hard, you could end up feeling anxious, which might make learning something new even more difficult. Choose activities that interest you and keep introducing new challenges, aiming to do something different once a week. As one 90-year-old woman proclaimed during one of my community memory talks, 'Stay curious!'

Specific programs dedicated to encouraging mental stimulation have become increasingly available in recent years. Some of these programs involve regular attendance over several weeks for repeated group training on particular memory or thinking tasks. Other online 'brain training' programs involve completing games and puzzles on a variety of devices. These programs typically improve people's performance on the trained tasks, although some researchers have questioned whether commercial brain training programs improve general, everyday memory function.[16] Recent studies have shown that participating in memory training programs can improve some untrained aspects of memory and thinking in healthy older people, but there is no evidence to show that these programs can prevent dementia.[17]

Attending skills training programs and doing online brain training can provide a fun and convenient way to include regular mental stimulation in your routine. Furthermore, many people report feeling more confident about their memory after taking part in these activities. As we have discussed in other chapters of this book, if you feel more positive about your memory, then you are often more willing to try new things, which in turn may help with building up 'brain resilience'.

Social engagement

Research examining risk factors for dementia has shown that being more socially isolated is associated with a greater likelihood of developing dementia.[18] There are many possible explanations for this finding. It could be that it is more difficult to take part in social activities when you have dementia. On the other hand, if you are not socially connected, this could increase your risk of depression, and reduce your mental stimulation, and both these factors have been associated with the development of dementia. It is difficult to be absolutely clear about what these research results mean, but specialists in dementia research recommend that we stay as socially connected as possible since this may have the potential to delay or reduce the risk of developing dementia. So spend time with your family, workmates, friends and neighbours. Participate regularly in book clubs, sports clubs, Senior Citizen's meetings or whatever appeals to you.

Diet

More and more research studies are examining the potential benefits of particular diets for maintaining brain health. Recent research on the 'Mediterranean diet' has shown that it is associated with better memory and thinking abilities in healthy older adults.[19] This diet includes a high intake of vegetables, fruit and fish, a low intake of meat and dairy products, and 1–2 glasses of wine per day.

Researchers investigating risk factors for dementia have found no definitive evidence that any particular diet or dietary supplement can prevent dementia.[20] However, it has become increasingly clear that obesity, diabetes, high blood pressure and high cholesterol are associated with the development of dementia, and what we eat is important for the management of these health issues. Emerging research has shown that people who follow a Mediterranean diet have fewer issues with diabetes and other health concerns that can cause damage to the blood vessels in the brain. It is important to review your eating habits with your doctor. If you would like to make changes to your diet, a dietitian can assist with a personalised nutrition plan.

Hearing

Dementia researchers have identified the management of hearing loss as an important factor when it comes to promoting 'brain resilience' to dementia,[21] although the evidence doesn't point towards a clear reason why hearing loss could decrease the brain's resilience to brain illnesses such as dementia. Scientists have proposed that there may be an indirect effect as reduced hearing ability often leads to less social engagement, which could even impact negatively on mood. The main message from the research is to have your hearing checked regularly, and wear hearing aids if they are recommended.

Sleep

Researchers have begun to investigate links between sleep, brain health and dementia. Sleep has been shown to be important for the formation of new memories.[22] In some studies, poor sleep quality was associated with reduced performance on memory and thinking tasks.[23] While more research on the importance of sleep in maintaining brain health is required, it is important to discuss any sleep difficulties with your doctor. Referral to a psychologist or sleep physician can help with enhancing sleep.

It is possible that sleep disordered breathing, sometimes called sleep apnoea, can cause changes in the brain that reduce the brain's resilience to dementia.[24] When people have sleep apnoea, they have difficulty breathing when they are asleep, which may be related to obstructions to the airway. Some research has suggested that sleep apnoea can cause damage to the brain due to changes in both the levels of oxygen and the flow of blood to the brain. Sleep apnoea is often associated with snoring and can cause daytime sleepiness. Tell your doctor if you suspect that you may have sleep disordered breathing, as there is simple, effective treatment available for this condition.

Putting your future brain health plan into action

So now you have gathered plenty of information for designing your personalised future brain health plan. Perhaps you have been to your doctor, seen one or more medical specialists, and identified some areas of your health and lifestyle that you would like to work on, so that you can keep your brain as healthy as possible, and potentially reduce your chances of developing dementia.

Life is a constant balancing act. Most of us know a lot about what we need to do to keep our bodies and minds healthy. Some of us like to live in the now and not worry about the future and how our body will age. Others spend time thinking towards the future and are willing to make changes to how they live now in an attempt to be healthier in the future. Taking the time to read this chapter probably means you are the type of person who is willing to commit to a future brain health plan in the hope that it will make a difference for your health as you get older.

Perhaps do for yourself what you would tell a close friend or family member to do. Would you advise them to spend time on their wellbeing now, in the hope that they would be healthier later? To introduce some preventive strategies now, so that they don't have to spend time when they are older, looking after a health problem that could possibly have been prevented? It's never too early or too late to make changes in order to maintain brain health—but your personalised future brain health plan won't work unless you put it into action!

It can be hard to make changes. We develop routines and it's often difficult to alter them. We think we don't have enough time to add new commitments to our already busy days. When it comes to making changes in your life to optimise your future brain health, you might find that you are already doing a lot of the things that have been recommended. You may just need to make a few small changes to the many positive steps you have already taken.

Of course there are only a certain number of hours in each day that you have to play with. Let's say you decide to focus on spending more time doing mentally stimulating activities. You are considering doing an hour of brain training on your computer or perhaps learning something new by reading a book. Before you commit to a new activity, it's important to think about the 'time trade-off'. You only have an hour of time in your day that you can dedicate to new activities aimed at maintaining brain health. If you spend that hour on your own, sitting down reading or doing brain training, then how will you make time for physical exercise and spending time with your family and friends? Perhaps, instead, you could stimulate your brain by learning about the history of your city or how to play golf? If you can squeeze in an hour doing a walking tour of your city with friends or having a golf lesson with your son, then you've covered the three main recommendations for building up your 'brain resilience' at once! You've combined mental stimulation, physical exercise and social engagement, and created a 'triple treat' for your future memory health!

When you think about it, many of the recommendations for your future brain health feed into each other. Making time for a 'triple treat' involving socialising, and exercise for your body and mind, can have a positive impact on other aspects of your life known to be important to brain health, such as your weight, and your mood. So go ahead, call a friend or family member and commit to a regular 'triple treat' for your brain. Think weekly exercise group, walking to a friend's house for a regular card playing session, or playing bowls at the club with your mates.

Further information

Your local dementia support organisation can provide further information and updates on the latest research on brain health and dementia prevention. Details of such support organisations are provided in the 'Resources' section at the end of this book. Your doctor or your local dementia support organisation can refer you to the latest clinical research trials that you may be able to participate in to assist with informing future generations about dementia prevention.

Key points   REDUCING THE RISK OF DEVELOPING DEMENTIA

- Scientists have identified multiple risk factors for dementia, including aspects of our physical and mental health, and lifestyle.
- Addressing these risk factors might have the potential to reduce the chance of developing dementia, or at least delay the onset of the symptoms of the disease.
- Health factors found to be associated with risk of developing dementia include high blood pressure, high cholesterol, diabetes, obesity, smoking, excessive alcohol consumption, depression, anxiety and stress.

- The latest research into reducing the risk of dementia has focused on ways we can build up 'brain resilience' to disease.
- Dementia researchers have promoted the importance of staying socially engaged, and taking part in regular physical exercise and mentally stimulating activities, with the aim of preventing or delaying the onset of dementia symptoms.

CHAPTER 6

Strategies for everyday memory

We all notice fluctuations in our ability to remember. We know that our memory can change as we get older (see Chapter 2 for a description of the way that memory changes with the ageing process). We also know that our physical and mental health, our attitude towards our memory, and the way we live our lives will affect our memory (see Chapters 3 and 4 for more detail about alterations in memory related to health, attitude and lifestyle). We can wisen up to changes in memory, and support our memory processing at times when we notice that it seems unreliable. This chapter outlines a variety of strategies to enhance everyday memory and make you feel more confident that you will remember to remember! Study and learning techniques are outlined in Chapter 7, and strategies for supporting memory during dementia are described in Chapters 8 and 9.

Dealing with memory change

Before you start to work on practical memory strategies, read the checklist of possible reasons for memory change at the end of

Chapter 3. Take the time to identify any factors that could be related to any change you are noticing in your memory at the moment and, if necessary, and possible, actively do something to work on these aspects of your health, attitude and lifestyle.

We know that for many older people, the main area of difficulty is getting new information into storage, and then getting it out quickly and completely when it is wanted. The most common memory lapses reported by older adults include remembering names, finding particular words and recalling something that happened recently. These inefficiencies in memory can be very frustrating, but we can learn to accommodate them in the same way as we learn to adapt to changes in our bodies as we get older. It's important to be patient with yourself. You don't need to remember everything or have a perfect memory. As mentioned in Chapter 1, forgetting is an important aspect of our memory system that prevents over-load. Prioritise your remembering and be realistic about the amount of information that you are able to recall. If you aim for a perfect memory, you could become stressed and anxious, which can end up making your memory worse. Instead, focus on remembering things that are important to you, and work on ways to promote your recall of these important details. Allow more time for mental processing: time for paying attention, for working on supportive strategies, and for practising recall of new information. Telling yourself to 'stay calm' will enhance recall, as panic and anxiety will just make remembering more difficult.

Recently, David returned to a memory skills group after a six-month break and said that the best memory strategy we had taught him was to 'stay calm'. He had worked hard at relaxing about his memory and putting less pressure on himself. Before this, he would berate himself for forgetting things and get worked up when people asked him to remember information. He constantly felt anxious about his failing memory and while people were telling him things that he had to remember, he wasn't able to focus on what they were saying because he was busy telling himself that he would forget because his memory was so poor. After teaching himself to 'stay calm' about remembering, David found that he was actually remembering more successfully.

Anne

I was driving to a friend's house a few days ago and I started to panic when I had a blank on how to get there. I remembered the words that you said to me. I said to myself 'stay calm'. I pulled over to the side of the road, took a few deep breaths, and eventually remembered how to get there.

Enza, 71

When I couldn't find my bike lights I made an effort to stay calm. I thought, what's the worst thing that could happen? I might have to buy another pair, but it's only money.

Kali, 54

I was at a school function and the mother of one of my son's friends approached me. I hadn't seen her for a long time and I searched my mind for her name, but it wouldn't come. I told myself to stay calm, and decided on another tactic. I said to her, 'Hello, it's Mandy, Jed's Mum'—and thankfully she returned the favour, by telling me her name!

Mandy, 48

Acknowledging and adapting to fluctuations in memory is important, but we can do more: we can also learn to make use of memory aids or strategies to enhance everyday recall and make us feel more in control. Using memory strategies can make you feel more positive about your ability to remember. If you think, 'I can remember this because I have a good strategy to help me remember', then you will begin to expect more from your memory. In turn, this could mean that your memory starts to work better for you because you are feeling more confident about remembering.

Most of us use memory strategies without realising it, for getting new information into the files, and also for getting old information out from that often overflowing mental filing cabinet which contains files for memories about family, friends, home, work, study and numerous other parts of our lives. Some strategies are simple, others quite involved.

Memory aids or strategies can be divided into two types. *Internal* memory strategies are the ones that come from within us and involve some sort of thinking: some mental manipulation. For example, to remember where you left your wallet, you might mentally retrace your steps since you last used it. *External* memory strategies involve using some sort of external aid to help memory— for example, a note pad for writing a shopping list, or a diary. They can also involve making changes to your external surroundings. For instance, you might put an item near the front door so that you remember to take it with you when you leave.

Let's now run through some examples of both internal and external strategies. Many of the following memory-wise tips come from talking to people about the strategies they use, and learning from their often creative and ingenious ideas. When you read through people's suggestions, you may be prompted to add your own. You might remember strategies that you haven't used for a while, or come up with variations on the ones included here. This list is by no means exhaustive—think of it as a starting point.

Internal memory strategies

The most common internal memory strategies involve three main features:

- focusing attention
- adding meaning to the information that you want to remember
- reducing the amount of information to be remembered.

These strategies are especially useful for older people, since paying attention to many aspects of information to be remembered is what many of us have difficulty with as we get older.

Some experts favour more elaborate techniques, such as mnemonics, so a few examples of these will be described, along with some discussion about their usefulness.

Focusing attention

We often say that we have 'forgotten' something, when what we really mean is that we didn't get it into the 'filing cabinet' in the first place because we didn't attend to it. Fluctuating attention is one of the most common explanations for fluctuating memory.

For instance, you might not remember what your friend was wearing at dinner the night before because you were paying attention to the interesting dinner guest sitting next to you, rather than to your friend's outfit; or you might not remember the name of the person you were introduced to before you made a speech because you did not pay attention to it—you were too anxious about the speech.

Of course, we can't expect to pay attention to everything in our environment. We all have a mental 'rubbish bin' where information that we don't need or don't want to know about gets dumped. We remember things that are important to us much better than things which we consider unimportant. For instance, some of us enjoy learning how to fix our own car, while others are happy for someone else to remember how to fix it!

When there is something important to remember and you want to focus your attention on it, aim to reduce any distractions. Put your phone away, ask people to be quiet, and stop multi-tasking. Focus on one thing at a time whenever possible.

I work in sales and marketing—so I've trained myself to learn people's names. I'm better doing this at work than socially. I focus and make a real effort to put it in, and rid myself of distractions. Socially, I don't make the effort; I let myself be distracted.

Ron, 63

How often do you meet someone for the first time, and not actually hear them say their name? Maybe you are nervous, or distracted by other thoughts, or things around you. You might be so focused on something happening in the background that you totally miss their name. The problem here is not one of forgetting, it is 'getting the information in'. If you slow down and listen carefully to the person's name when you first meet them, you will have a better chance of remembering it later. If you don't hear the name, don't be afraid to say, 'I didn't hear your name clearly.'

In general, it is helpful to make a *conscious effort* to attend to the key aspects of the new information you want to get into your memory files, such as the name of a person that you are being introduced to. Paying attention to paying attention also helps when it comes to remembering where you have put things, such as your keys, wallet or even your car!

The best way for me to remember where my car is located in a large car park is to concentrate on landmarks close to my car, like the floor number, or the colour of a nearby feature. I also look behind me as I am walking away from my car, and concentrate on how my car, and the landmarks around it, will look when I come back to it.
Mary, 81

One of my friends shared her confusion at carefully remembering the '8' sign beside her car, and on returning to the '8' sign, realised they were speed signs, which were everywhere . . . and on every floor!
Delys, when she was in her sixties

Rehearsal and repetition
Rehearsal and repetition are common strategies which help us to focus attention. Repetition involves repeating information out loud, whereas rehearsal is done in our heads.

For many of us, rehearsal and repetition are good strategies for remembering names. It can help even more if we stage the timing of our mental rehearsals. To do this, you gradually increase the amount of time between rehearsals. You might even rehearse the information again the next day.

I find that the best way for me to remember someone's name is to repeat it to myself three times after I have heard it.
Angela, 34

Reinforcing rehearsal with repetition is useful. You can ask someone to repeat their name by saying, for example, 'Would you mind telling me your name again, I would like to get it right', 'Could you spell your name?', or, 'How do you pronounce your name correctly?' People are often pleased that you are making an effort to learn their name.

I decided to try out this technique when I was at work, and I couldn't recall the surname of a colleague who had recently joined our team. I had to write her name on a form, so I needed to find it out quickly. I thought I was being very clever when I asked her, 'Sue, how do you spell your surname?' as I went to write it on the form. She looked at me with a bemused expression, and spelt out 'S m i t h'!
Anne, when I was in my forties

Using a person's name in the ensuing conversation often makes it easier to remember later on.

My trouble is with concentration. When I meet someone, I say, 'Nice to meet you, Anne', and then later I say their name again during our conversation, and again when I say goodbye. If I say the name repeatedly, it helps me to remember it.
Leo, 70

Remember learning poems at school? We did this by repeating them over and over again until they were memorised. Some say this is a great way to remember jokes. Tell the joke to someone else straight away—tell it on as many different occasions as possible.

Do you ever wonder whether you have turned the iron or the oven off, or shut a window? Maybe you wonder if you locked a door when you left the house. Some people suggest that it helps to say out loud what you are doing at the time, so you might say, 'I've turned the iron off' to yourself or to someone else. Next time you walk into a friend's house and put your keys and wallet down, pause and say to your friend, 'I have put my keys and wallet on your kitchen bench', and this will make it easier to find them when you go to leave. Sometimes the simple act of talking can increase your attention enough to make you remember what you have done or not done.

Adding meaning

As we discussed in Chapter 1, scientists believe that how well we remember something depends on how deeply we process the information. If we attend to as many aspects as possible of the information to be remembered, then this 'deep' processing should help us to remember it later.

Deliberately being alert to, and using, the senses can help— for example, to remember a particular rose, focus on feeling its thorns, seeing its colour and shape, smelling its fragrance, while saying its name. We all learn from a very early age to associate certain memories with smell, taste, sound, sight, touch and movement. Certain people, for instance chefs and wine judges, seem to be especially good at a particular type of sense memory.

Some say that it also helps to *make a judgement* about what we are wanting to remember. Do you like it or not? How does it make you feel? Or you can make a conscious link with a piece of information already stored. You might want to think about how unusual a person's name is, or how the name reminds you of someone you knew when you were younger. You could also see what it looks like when it is written down. Can you get a special meaning from the name? For instance, if you can remember that your friend's children both have names that start with L, you might find it easier to recall that the names are Luke and Louise when you see them next.

Common techniques that add meaning to the information to be remembered are associating and visualising. Some people use rhymes or acrostics to add meaning in a particular way. Let's run through these techniques now.

Making associations

Associating new information with something that we already know well is one way to add meaning to what we want to remember. It is normal to have some trouble with putting names to faces as we get older. Typically, we can't get the name out quickly and when we need to use it, but later on, usually when we don't need to use the name, it pops into our heads. This is an example of 'slowed recall'—a common age-related change. We can remember the name, but it takes longer to 'get it out' of memory storage than it used to do when we were younger. When you stop to think about it, it's no wonder that we have difficulty remembering names—they are just random words, without any meaning. If we make an effort to add meaning to names when we learn them, then it may become easier to recall the name later when we need it. You will probably find that if you connect or associate a name you have just heard with someone who has the same name and whom you know well, then the name is easier to remember. You might sometimes associate the new name with a famous personality, too!

Souad didn't think that using association was going to work for her when I suggested this technique to help her remember her neighbour's name. She was so pleased when she reported back to me that she had worked out that her neighbour's name 'Sofia' was the same as the name of the street that a good friend lives in, and that this association had given her success with recalling the name!

Anne

A friend told me that she remembered the name of a man she met called Grant, by thinking of Government Grant, because he worked for the public service.

Serge, 60

Another way to associate information is to connect something you want to remember to do with something that happens regularly around the same time. For example, you might associate taking your medication with mealtimes, or with cleaning your teeth at night. Thus, something that you already do on a regular basis will trigger your memory for something else that you have to do.

Association is also useful to increase our knowledge in a certain area. The more you know about a particular thing or issue, the easier it is to learn more about it. This is because you have more memory files on which that knowledge is based, and thus it is easier to make new associations.

I'm very good at remembering the names of trees since I've got a background in forestry—but things that don't interest me, like fish for example, I simply don't recall.

Ross, 72

In this way, getting new information into our files can be easier because we have a good range of knowledge stored in the past to link new ideas to. Filing is easier. We don't have to create a new folder each time, because we can put new files into already well-established folders.

The more I learn about plant names, the easier it is for me to remember new ones. The other day I saw a plant that I wanted to buy, so I looked up its botanical name. It was a Wattle, and I already knew that 'acacia' was the term for Wattle. It had purple growth tips, and I knew the word for that is 'purpurea'. The only new part that I had to remember was 'Baileyana'. This was easy because I have a friend named 'Anna Bailey'.

If I hadn't known the terms for 'wattle' and 'purple', then I would have needed to remember three words, instead of just one!
Dianne, 41

As mentioned in Chapter 2, older people can draw on their life skills and developed wisdom to ensure effective learning. Experts in particular fields can use association to their advantage so that they can perform as well as, if not better than, younger novices who may be motivated and able to think fast.

Using associations can also help us get information *out* of our storage files; we can use them as cues. One type of cueing strategy that we often use is called a 'logical search'. This can be useful for those frustrating 'tip of the tongue' experiences, when we know that we have a word or name somewhere in our storage files, but cannot get it out when we want it! Especially difficult are proper names—like names of authors, actors, or hotels that you have visited. In this situation, a logical search would involve running through the letters of the alphabet, and thinking of possible names or words that begin with each letter.

People may also use sounds or smells to cue for information from a storage file. As outlined in Chapter 1, the use of 'filing tabs' in our memory filing cabinet can assist us in locating a particular file when we want it. Who you were with, where you were standing and the time of the day when you were told the name of a particular rose may help you to recall it when someone admires it in your garden next spring!

Contextual cues are also useful for 'tip of the tongue' experiences. Many people find that it helps to think of the situation where they first remembered the name or word. For remembering a name, you could think about where you last saw the person and any details about your conversation. Some say it is also helpful to think about the mood you were in. Recreating the context in your mind can make it easier to re-establish some connections, and get the word or name out of your storage files.

I had been trying for a long time to remember the family name of a girl I went to school with, over 50 years ago. Usually I take great pride in my ability to remember names, but this one was getting to me. It was funny how I did eventually come to remember the name. I visualised the area where I grew up, and where my school was. All of a sudden it came to me: the name that I had been searching for jumped back into my mind all of its own.

Brian, 74

The use of action or location cues has also been suggested to help remember the location of something that is lost (e.g. your wallet). You can mentally retrace your steps: go through step by step what you did, where you were after that, and where you last saw the thing. For instance, 'Where did I put the mail?—I collected it from the letter box, I came inside, I put my keys on the sideboard, I went into the kitchen to put the milk in the fridge . . . Aaaah! I left the mail on top of the fridge.' It can also help to actually return to the last place that you were in.

Sometimes I walk into a room and forget what I was going to say. If I go back to where I came from, voilà!—the words that I was going to say miraculously appear.

Graham, 91

If you can't remember where you have put something, you could pretend that you are putting the thing away for the first time and think of the likely places you would put it. How many of us go into a room to get something and forget what we've gone in to get! If you find yourself in this situation, you could think back, or actually go back, to the place where you first had that thought.

Visualising

Another way to process information at a 'deeper' level and add meaning to it is to visualise it—to picture something in your mind, or create an image of the thing to be remembered. Some people say that the more unusual or funny the image, the more they will remember it. For some people, visualisation is a strong tool that can provide a very quick way of remembering. The power of visualisation is reflected in the old Chinese proverb, 'One seeing is worth ten thousand tellings'—or the modern saying, 'A picture is worth a thousand words.'

I remember my friend Vee Lyn by imagining her playing the violin!
Valerie, 67

Whenever I park my car in a multi-storey car park, I look around for landmarks that I can visualise to help me remember where it is. There is usually a number or a letter, or even a colour that stands out. On a recent holiday in Darwin, the supermarket car park had paintings of animals to mark different sections. It was so easy to remember that my car was parked in the crocodile aisle!
Winston, 77

I have one memory trick that I was taught in primary school, yet whenever I tell anyone they look at me as if I'm crazy. I was told that an easy way to remember how to spell accommodation was to imagine booking two double rooms—hence the double 'c' and the double 'm'. Silly? It works for me!
Clare, 53

Audrey was having difficulty recalling the names of her new neighbour's two little girls, Ruby and Charley. When I suggested that she think of a visual image to help her remember the names, she came up with a vision from the film *Charlie and the Chocolate Factory*, where the chocolate lake was filled with a new variety of chocolate, called 'Ruby' chocolate. Next time she saw the girls, she visualised the ruby red chocolate lake, and proudly came up with both girls' names!
Anne

Spaced recall

Once you have added meaning to a name by using association or visualisation, you can then practise recall of the name to help get the name into memory storage, and make it more readily accessible when you need it next. This process is sometimes called 'spaced recall'. Think of what you do when you learn a new PIN (personal identification number) for banking. You rehearse the number a few times, you use the PIN on the same day, and then again a few days later. By the time you have recalled the number regularly for a few months, it comes automatically to you. This is how spaced recall works. This technique works well for learning names, passwords and numbers, especially when combined with added meaning from association and/or visualisation. For example, you can choose a PIN or password that relates to well-stored knowledge from your past, such as an old phone number, address or car registration number. It is a process that takes some time, but sometimes it is worth taking the time to learn something successfully, especially information that you need to know, but have been unable to master.

Why don't you challenge yourself to learn a name—one that always eludes you. Write the name down and decide on a way to make the name more meaningful. Put some effort in and process the name as deeply as you can. Now cover the name with your hand and say the name out loud. Recall the name again in a few minutes and then a few hours. Recall the name the next day as well. The more that you recall the name from your memory storage, the more likely that it will come out when you see the person next. After you have successfully remembered this name that has been escaping you for so long, you will feel much more positive about your memory for names.

I kept having difficulty recalling the dog breed name Rottweiler. So I decided I would work on this. First I came up with a visual association for the word. I imagined a big black Rottweiler with wheels instead of feet! I typed a prompt question into the reminders section of my

phone ('What is the name of the big black dog?') and I programmed my reminder to come up once a month. Now my phone comes up with my prompt question once a month and I practise recalling the word. I think I've finally ironed out this glitch in my recall system!
Saskia, 59

Rhymes

Many of us can remember nursery rhymes from our childhood days. Making a rhyme about information to be remembered is another internal strategy which involves adding meaning to the information to be remembered.

One common early learned rhyme is: 'Thirty days hath September, April, June, and November. All the rest have 31, except February alone, which has 28 days clear, and 29 days each leap year'—and the not-so-well-known version: 'Thirty days hath September, all the rest I don't remember'! Some people use another version of this. If you say the months of the year with the aid of your trusty knuckle-bones, you will always know how many days each month has. Put your closed fists together, to make a row of knuckles. Start with January, by touching the knuckle furthest to the left. February is the space between the knuckles. March is the next knuckle, and so on. July and August both fall on knuckles—there is no space between them. All the months that fall on a knuckle have 31 days.

'I before e except after c' is another rhyme in common use by English speakers, although this one is not 100 per cent reliable!

Acrostics

Acrostics are sometimes used to add meaning to information that we want to remember. To do this, the first letter of each word on a list is used to make up a sentence.

Anyone who has learned music is probably familiar with the following acrostics: 'Every Good Boy Deserves Fruit' (the lines of the treble staff: E, G, B, D, F), and 'All Cows Eat Grass' (the notes on the spaces of the bass staff: A, C, E, G).

Do you know what this acrostic is used to remember: 'Richard Of York Gains Battles In Vain'?

Yes—it's the colours of the rainbow: Red, Orange, Yellow, Green, Blue, Indigo, Violet.

Of course, 'My dear Aunt Sally' helps us to remember the mathematical order of operations—multiply or divide before you add or subtract.

Reducing the amount of information to be remembered

Earlier we mentioned that internal strategies can assist us by reducing the amount of information we have to get into our storage files. There are many ways of doing this—for instance grouping and acronyms.

Grouping

This involves grouping or 'chunking' bits of information together. Many of us do this when we learn new phone numbers. We might split the phone number into two or three parts. Association can also be used to add further meaning.

Our local Seniors Information phone number is 1300 135090. I remember it in chunks, 1300 13 50 90. The 50 and 90 at the end is easy to remember. I think of seniors ranging in age from 50 to 90. Then I just need to remember 1300 and to repeat the first two digits of 1300 again before the seniors' age range.
Sonia, 77

You might like to use grouping, association and spaced recall to learn a family member or close friend's mobile phone number. How proud will you feel when you can recall this number at a time of need, perhaps when your phone is out of battery and you can't rely on your phone's memory, but instead can rely on your own memory!

Some people remember a list of things to buy at the shops by grouping similar items together. Then they can use the categories of items to help remember each item. Think back to the shopping list that you recalled in Chapter 1:

Milk
Soap
Apples
Bananas
Yoghurt
Shampoo
Lemons
Cheese
Toothpaste

Did you recall the items by grouping them? If you were not able to write down a list to take with you, then it might help if you group items into categories. How would you group these items? When you get to the supermarket, you then have to recall the categories, and what was in each of them.

'What *fruit* do I need to buy? Of course, it was apples, bananas and lemons. And what about the *dairy produce*? Yes, it was milk, yoghurt and cheese. Now the last thing, *bathroom products*—what were they? Um, soap, shampoo and toothpaste.'

Acronyms

Acronyms are another way of reducing the amount of information to be remembered. You take the first letter of each word in a list and use these initial letters to make up a new word.

Many of you will be familiar with 'ROY G BIV' as a way to remember the colours of the rainbow in order. All you have to do is run through each letter, and recall what each letter stands for— Red, Orange, Yellow, Green, Blue, Indigo, Violet.

'DRS ABCD' helps us to recall 'Danger, Response, Send for help, Airway, Breathing, Compression, Defibrillation' in times of emergency. 'RICE' helps us to remember that 'Rest, Ice, Compression and Elevation' are important after any injury.

Maybe this prompts you to think of some acronyms that you have found useful. People are able to be creative with acronyms in using a well-known word to remember something new. For instance, my name is Anne and I am learning the routine for answering telephone calls at my new office; I remember A for 'answer', N for 'number', N for 'name' and E for 'extension'.

Mnemonics

The word 'mnemonic' comes to us from Greek mythology. The goddess of memory was called Mnemosyne. Books or training courses for 'improving your memory' often describe mnemonic (pronounced nee-mon-ick, with the stress on 'mon') techniques. While mnemonic strategies can be fun, many are quite complex and take time to learn. These more elaborate techniques are often difficult to apply in everyday situations. Here are a few examples to test out.

Method of loci

This mnemonic strategy uses visual association of objects with a predetermined set of locations. Let's say you want to impress your friends by remembering that nine-item list of shopping items in a particular order. To do this you could imagine walking through your house, and visually associate the nine items on the list with nine locations in your house.

So you might associate the first item, *milk*, with the front door. You could imagine opening the *front door* to collect the milk after it has been delivered. The second item was *soap*, and you might imagine the soap on your *hall table*. You then continue to imagine walking through your house, associating each item with particular locations, in the order that you would see these locations as you walk through your house. When you need to recall the list of items, you take a mental trip through your house. You imagine each item sitting in its location and reel off the list. Wow—how clever!

This technique is fine for lists of words. But it is not very often that many of us need to remember a list of words in a particular order. When you try the technique with everyday remembering, such as lists of names of people, it can be more difficult to visualise, which can make this mnemonic technique even more complex.

Peg-word method

Another mnemonic technique to test out is also a 'seeing in your mind's eye', or visualisation method, called the peg-word method. The idea here is to visually associate the objects on your shopping list with another list of words, which are remembered using a rhyme.

You will first need to learn the following rhyme:

1 is a bun
2 is a shoe
3 is a tree
4 is a door
5 is a hive
6 is sticks
7 is heaven
8 is a gate
9 is a vine
10 is a hen

You can see that each number is associated with a rhyming word that can be transformed into a mental picture or image. For this technique, you will associate the first word from the list, that is *milk*, with a *bun*. You might visualise a bun going soggy because it has milk spilt all over it. You continue on. The second word *soap* is associated with *shoe*. What image could you create to link these two? When you want to recall the list, you recite each line of the rhyme one by one, and remember the vivid image that you have created to link the two objects.

Some people use these elaborate internal techniques, which they have practised and perfected, to learn amazing amounts of information. Unfortunately, being able to remember 100 digits after only hearing them once, or learning a list of 10 phone numbers in 10 minutes, does not mean that you will be able to remember where you put your wallet, when to turn the sprinkler off, or that the saucepan may boil dry if not checked!

Complex mnemonic strategies can be useful if you are studying for exams or learning a list of facts or a set of information, but they do not improve your memory overall, and are generally used to recall things that most of us do not commonly need to remember in our everyday routine. Moreover, they are often not user-friendly and can require a great deal of effort and time for success. You also have to 'remember' the details of how to apply the strategy, and if you are experiencing difficulty with getting new information into storage, this could be a problem. When you have to remember a list of nine items to buy at the supermarket, wouldn't it be much easier to write them down, and take the list with you?

External memory strategies

External memory strategies involve the use of some sort of external aid, like a diary or smartphone, or making changes to your external surroundings to support memory. Common external strategies involve writing things down, putting something in a special place, alarms and technical devices, and asking someone to remind you.

External strategies work best when we are **organised.** Someone with a good memory is usually a well-organised person, but it is also true that a well-organised person has more chance of remembering well. It is often at times when we are disorganised that we begin to wonder about our memory—when we are busy, rushed, stressed, in unfamiliar places, on holiday, moving house or without assistance at work. At times like these, you might keep very good notes in your diary, but forget to look at your notes at the right time, or even worse, forget to take your diary with you when you need it. Or you might have written a detailed shopping list, but not be able to find it anywhere.

The strategies or devices that become part of your daily habits and **routine** will be the most beneficial. They will reduce the demand on your memory. If you use a diary, for example, it helps to make checking your diary something that you do at the start of every day—part of your routine in the morning, or the last thing that you do that day. You can keep your shopping list in a designated place—for example, attached to the fridge in your kitchen. If you have special places for things, make sure that you put them back in that place when you've finished with them!

If you are really into routine, you could even try to do things at set times of the day, or on set days of the week. For instance, the rubbish has to be put out on Mondays, your tablets need to be taken straight after breakfast each day, and your weekly luxury massage is on a Thursday. This helps to take the load off memory even more.

It's a good idea to act immediately whenever possible, or **do it now!** When you think 'I must water that plant', and it is possible at the time—water it right then; then there's no need to remember it later. Similarly, use your memory aids as soon as possible— if you are cooking and use the last of the sugar, write down on your shopping list at the time that you need sugar next time you do the shopping. Or if you are lying in bed at night and think, 'I must remember to get those tablets from the chemist tomorrow', write this down on tomorrow's date in your diary, or on a piece of paper that you keep by the bed, or get up and put the prescription by the front door. Many people forget these sleepy inspirations by morning. Remembering to remember to do something is especially difficult when we are unwell, stressed or overwhelmed. During times like these, capture your ideas as soon as you think of them. Type a reminder into your phone or write in your diary what you need to do on a particular day or at a specific time.

I am so busy at the moment it's ridiculous. I find that if I don't write something down at the time that I think about it—I completely forget about it later. My diary is my lifeline! I don't know what I'd do without it.
Russell, 56

I'm always leaving things behind or forgetting to take something I intend to. What I do now is, as soon as I think of it, put the item somewhere to remind me later. I might put a book in the car when I know I have to return it to the library the next day, or put letters that I have to post on the hall floor.
Jyoti, 76

After moving into the retirement village a few weeks ago, I am feeling exhausted and I keep forgetting the names of all the new people I am meeting. As soon as I walked in the door after our village book club last night, I wrote down the names of the new people that I had met. Now I can read their names before book club next week, and have more chance of remembering them.
Stella, 69

Many people use external strategies as a 'back-up' system for their memory. The very process of putting the back-up system into action makes us focus attention on the thing to be remembered, so we often don't have to use the system—but it is reassuring to know that it is there. For example, the process of writing something down on a calendar might make it easier to recall that information later on and we might not have to refer to the calendar at all. Writing out a shopping list helps us in remembering what we wanted to buy—this is especially useful when we get to the shop and find we have left the list at home. And don't we feel proud of our achievement when we get home and check the list to find we got everything!

My analogy for memory is a 50-cent piece on jelly. The longer you leave the 50 cents there, the stronger the imprint it makes on the jelly. That's how I think about memory. When I meet someone, I say their

name a few times whilst I'm talking to them, so the name makes an impression on my memory, like the 50 cents on the jelly. It's the same with shopping lists. If I take the time to write a list, I don't need to take it with me because I have impressed the information onto my memory.
Nic, 73

Writing things down
If I write it down, I don't have to waste my time remembering it.
Jacob, 49

There aren't many of us who haven't written something down so that we will remember it later. People use written memory aids for remembering just about anything!

Where something is located
Writing things down helps us remember where things are. We label folders, so that we know what is in them. We label drawers of filing cabinets for the same reason. Sometimes it would be very useful to have a few more labels around the home!

I got so sick of rearranging the linen press at our holiday house that I decided to write labels on each shelf. Now people who stay there know which size sheets go on which shelf! I wish I had got my black marker pen out earlier!
Moira, 55

Some people write down the level that their car is parked on when it is in a multi-storey car park. You can write it on your ticket if you take it with you, in your diary or phone or perhaps resort to the back of your hand!

For that odd occasion when you do leave something behind, some suggest that you write or engrave your name and address for return on things that you might leave around, such as your umbrella, book, glasses or handbag.

Something that you have to do

People use diaries or calendars to help them to remember social events, appointments, medication for pets, and other important things to do. Many people use digital diaries and reminder systems on technical devices. Either system works—it's just a matter of choosing a written reminder system that suits you.

At a parent information night at my son's school when he was in Grade 6, his teacher handed out student planners to the class. She said, 'I want you to get into the habit of using these planners because the more organised you are with your planners, the more organised you will be in here', pointing to her head!
Anne

Calendars are often used as 'social planners'. If something is written on the household calendar, then everyone in the house knows about it, which can prevent double-booking. It is important to hang the calendar in a place where everyone will see it and to look at it regularly. Next to the phone, on the fridge or in the kitchen are all good locations.

My husband is always up-to-date on our social plans now—I've hung the calendar in the toilet!
Varinder, 68

When I was at work I never had to keep a diary, as my personal assistant did this for me. Now that I'm retired, I'm finding it hard to keep on top of all my social engagements and appointments. I think I'm going to have to be my own personal assistant now, and buy a diary!
Dennis, 72

A diary is useful if you are often on the move, as you can take it with you wherever you go. It helps to get into the habit of checking your diary as part of your daily routine.

> 'Memory is the diary that we all carry about with us.'
>
> Oscar Wilde, 1895

A diary that allows space for a list of things to do is doubly useful. Or you might want to use a separate notebook as a compilation of your 'to do' lists and future plans.

I write all my bright ideas in a notebook that sits on my desk. I want to renovate my garden this spring, so I have a few pages where I write down ideas for plants and the conditions that each plant likes to grow in. When I think of a good idea for a gift for one of my grandchildren, I write that down too. If I write the ideas down, I'm more likely to follow up on them.
Gail, 80

Keep your reminder system as streamlined as possible. If you write reminders in too many different spots, you might forget where you have written the reminder! Whiteboards or blackboards in strategic places are sometimes preferred over pieces of paper that tend to get lost. Leaving your notes in attention-grabbing places can often jog your memory about something that has to be done. Sticky 'Post-it' notes must have been designed for exactly this purpose. Their bright colour makes them stand out—but beware, they have been known to fall off!

I put a post-it note around my front door key to remind me to do something when I get home.
Judith, 87

What to take with you
When you are about to go on holiday you are usually very busy, tying up all those loose ends before you go. It can be very helpful

to write down, not only what you have to get done, but also what you have to take with you. If you tick off each item on the list as you pack it, and take a final look at the list before you leave home, then you are more likely to remember everything you need.

We have a holiday list for the family which we keep in a special drawer and pull out each time we go away.
Jackie, 62

What to buy
We all have different ways of compiling a shopping list, and it is something that most of us do regularly. Some people hang a list in their kitchen, and write things on it as they discover they need them. Others compile a list just before they go shopping. Some people have a pre-printed list of commonly needed items, and tick each one as needed. Others are even more organised . . .

I have a very analytical mind and like to list my weekly grocery shopping in the same order as the rows of the supermarket. This saves me time and having to retrace my steps, to go back to aisle 5 to get the olives, etc. The system worked well until a decision was made to enlarge and remodel the store. It quite threw me out and I didn't know whether I was Arthur or Martha for several weeks.
Terry, 68

What people tell you
One of the most common times that we have to remember what people tell us is when we take a phone message. For this, it is useful to have a pad by the phone. It is even more useful to have a pen there, too—one that works—preferably attached to the pad.

Many people carry a notebook with them at all times. This can be useful for jotting down things that people tell you and that you will want to remember later—good books, nice wines, names of plants that you admire, new phone numbers and addresses—the list goes on! Some people find it helpful to take notes when they visit the doctor. It can be useful to prepare a list of what you want to talk about, and also to note any particular suggestions that the doctor outlines. It is also handy to keep a notepad in the car.

If you attend lectures or seminars, take notes to help remember what was said. You will need to keep track of where you keep the notes, and summarising key points later or telling someone about the presentation will help to consolidate the memories. After someone has shown you how to use a new household appliance, such as a TV remote control, you can write down step-by-step instructions, and even stick them to the appliance. See Chapter 7 for more techniques for learning how to use anything new.

Address books and birthday books are another example of written memory aids. Not many of us are able to remember all our friends' and colleagues' names, addresses, phone numbers and birthdays without looking them up.

Names

Written memory strategies can be very useful when it comes to remembering people's names.

I work in marketing, and I think it's important to address people by their names. I have a pad by the phone. When someone says who they are, I immediately write down their name. Then I can say goodbye, using their name. It also gives me a handy record of whom I have spoken to during the day.

Paula, 46

I started a new job in sales six weeks ago and I've had to learn a lot of new names of staff and customers. I go to ring someone, and I can't remember their name to call them. I end up scrolling through my contact list on my phone until I finally recognise the name of the person and then I can call them.

Oanh, 39

Written name tags are worn by staff in hospitals and are often used at social gatherings. Name tags work best if they are worn high on your body, and are in large print, so that people can readily read the name. Wouldn't it be convenient if we all had name badges stuck to our foreheads!

Some organised people keep a list of the names of people they are likely to see at a semi-regular meeting, and read through the list as preparation before going to the meeting.

Before I go to a work meeting, I do some preparation. I get my papers out and I go through everyone's names and then I'm more likely to remember them at the meeting.
Dino, 72

Record-keeping
When you think about it, written memory strategies play a big part in our memory of things past, in literature and history.

On a personal level, we write things down in diaries (for that future autobiography!), photo albums (written captions), travel diaries and 'baby milestones' books. We may want to retain the details of a recipe we created, or one a friend tells us. Written records of past financial accounts are often consulted. Some people keep written records of presents they have given people, and lists of people they send Christmas cards to each year.

I've done it twice now—given the same present to my mother and my brother two years in a row. It was such a good idea, that I thought of it again! Mum loves scarves, and Hugh loves books about gardening. Needless to say, I now keep a book in which I laboriously list the presents that I give to people each year.
Cath, 44

At work many people record daily statistics of regularly completed activities. Remembering to use the travel log book in the car for recording kilometres driven is essential for income-tax claims for some working people.

Putting something in a special place

Where something is located

Some people have set places in their home or workplace for specific things that they use, especially things that they use regularly. Wouldn't it be great to always know where your keys, your wallet and your glasses are?

When you first work out the special place to store objects, it can be helpful if you think of it, and where you have put it, at regular intervals afterwards. If you make these intervals a little longer each time, it can help reinforce your memory of where something is stored.

Colour can be used to make the location and the object more visible. Buy brightly coloured versions of things such as keys and wallets, or store them in colourful bowls or boxes.

It's important that I shut the roller door on my garage each day, but I'd been finding it hard to find the little black zapper that I have to press to operate the door. This week I put the zapper into a little red purse that I keep on the kitchen bench with my keys, and now I can find it more easily.

Goya, 69

It helps if you store an object in a function-related spot. For example, many people store their keys near the front door of their house. This makes sense because most of us pick up our keys as we leave the house, and it is easy to put them back there when we return.

This brings up an important point. When you've finished with something, make sure that you return it to its special location, ready for the next time that you are wondering where it is.

I've worked out the best place to keep my glasses. Around my neck! Since I've attached them to a chain and worn them around my neck, I've spent a lot less time searching for my glasses.

Dora, 84

We have so many electrical cords in our house for all the different devices—charger cords, connecting cords and cords for the camera to put the photos onto the computer. I decided to get organised. On the inside of a cupboard I hung a clear plastic divider that is designed for storing pairs of shoes. I labelled each compartment for a particular device, and put the labelled cord for each device neatly inside the compartment. I feel so proud of myself now when I can quickly select the right cord for the job!

Philomena, 51

I was always losing my ticket in car parks. Then I discovered that the visor on the windscreen had a little strap on it. Now I always know where my car park ticket is because as soon as I get it, I put it under the strap on my car visor.

Bill, 71

Something that you have to do

If you put something in a special place, where it is visible, then it will act as a reminder to do something. You are more likely to act on that reminder if you see it. How many times have you heard someone say, 'Out of sight, out of mind'? For example, if you put the birthday card that you have bought for a friend on the kitchen bench, it will help you to remember to write it.

I was at my parents' house for dinner. The news was on TV and I was watching a story about a house fire, where two children had died. I suddenly remembered that I had forgotten to turn off my perfumed oil-burner candle that was sitting on my desk, surrounded by papers. I panicked and I could feel my heart thumping in my chest. 'Oh no—our house could be in flames, and it's all my fault.' My fear was exacerbated by my recollection of another news story about a house fire caused by someone leaving their oil burner on. I rang our neighbour—who, thankfully, informed me that the house was still standing when she had driven past it five minutes previously. Since then, I've put the oil burner by the study door. Now I can't help but see it—and of course blow the candle out—before I leave the room!

Zara, 38

If you need to remember to take certain medications, you can put them near the thing that acts as your memory trigger. For instance, if you take your tablets after you brush your teeth, put them near the toothpaste. If you take them with meals, put them somewhere obvious in the kitchen. If you have several medications to take at various times throughout the day, it can be helpful to keep them in a dosette box. This is a plastic box, divided up like a grid into compartments for the days of the week, with different time slots. You can sort your tablets into this box, which serves as a reminder to take the tablets, and also helps to keep track of the last time that you took them. Many people use homemade variations on this theme, or arrange for special blister packs to be made up by their local pharmacist.

Some people find it useful to have a reminder that's in view most of the time, or that they can't avoid seeing. There are many different ways to do this, including putting a ring on a different finger, putting a knot in your handkerchief, putting a rubber band on your wrist, and putting your watch on the opposite wrist.

My physiotherapist told me to put a fluoro-coloured dot sticker in places that I go regularly throughout the day, such as the toilet, the car and the kitchen pantry. He said that every time I see the coloured dot, I have to stop and do my exercises!

Trish, 62

What to take with you

Some people have a special place, like the hall table near their front door, for things they need to take with them each day. Others create an obstacle at the front door with the object they need to take with them, so they can't forget it! The front door is also a useful place to put a 'sticky note' telling you what to remember to take with you.

Another option is to put what you want to take with you straight into your bag or briefcase. It helps to do this as soon as you think of it.

At work, I often used to leave my food shopping in the fridge, instead of taking it home at the end of the day. Someone gave me a great tip. If you put your car keys in the fridge with the food, you can't leave work without it! I use this idea to remember lots of things—I just put my car keys with whatever I need to remember to collect.

Malcolm, 57

Our supermarket no longer provides plastic bags to take your shopping home in, so that means I have to remember to take my own bags or I have nothing to transport my food home in. I keep some cloth bags in the passenger seat of my car, and I also keep a lightweight fabric bag within my handbag just in case I forget to take the cloth bags into the supermarket with me.

Mia, 81

It can be very frustrating when you leave your bag or umbrella somewhere, especially on public transport. One idea is to put the handle of these items around your wrist, so that they are attached to you, and you will notice them when you get up to leave.

Where you are up to in a book

Placing a bookmark in a book is a popular way of reminding ourselves where we left off the last time we were reading it. A bookmark can be a simple scrap of paper, or a fancy one made of exquisite embossed leather. Or you might be lucky enough to have a ribbon attached to the book—which has the added advantage that you don't have to spend time looking for it.

Alarms and technical devices

Technical devices are an essential part of everyday life, and most of us use some sort of computer or phone. We might search the internet for information, send email messages or make use of one of the new applications ('apps') that seem to be developed on an almost daily basis to help us negotiate everyday life.

Many of us are reluctant to use new technology. Some older people carry their mobile phone in case of emergency, and may not have learned how to send and receive text messages, let alone use the reminder function. When you haven't grown up with computers and mobile phones, you sometimes feel nervous about learning how to use them. It is worth trying to overcome this hesitancy about new technology because our phones and computers can serve as valuable memory support systems. They are especially helpful with remembering what we have to do, and where we have put things. (For practical strategies for learning how to use new devices, see Chapter 7.)

Something that you have to do

Most phones and computers have a calendar or reminder function where you can type in what you need to remember at a specific time on a particular day. Make sure you type in full what the reminder is for, as a one-word reminder may not make any sense to you when it flashes up in a few weeks' time! When the allotted time arrives, your phone will make a noise and your reminder will come up on the screen for you to read. Some location-based systems will provide a reminder when you're near a particular location, and may provide details of how long it will take you to get to your appointment from your current location.

Timely prompts like these can help us remember a whole range of things, such as attending an appointment, taking medication, or taking a blood sugar reading at a particular time. If the reminder comes at a time when we are not able to complete the task, many apps allow you to 'snooze' the reminder, and the reminder is repeated again later to make sure you don't forget what you planned to do.

Some people prefer to use an electronic pill reminder system rather than a computer or phone reminder system to assist with taking medication. These systems are a combination of a multi-compartment dosette box and an electronic alarm system. You can program these medication dispensers to sound an alarm and open the lid of a particular compartment on a specified day and time. Reminder alarms usually continue to sound until the medication is taken.

If you are using an app on your device to remind you about an appointment or a birthday, it may be best to program the alarm to come on before the event, so that you have time to get ready for it. Digital calendars allow you to share or 'synchronise' your calendar with others, so as to create a streamlined family diary. They also have a handy 'search' function.

You can use your smartphone to send a text message to yourself as a reminder, or perhaps to a friend or relative. If you have provided your mobile phone number, you will probably receive a variety of text reminders from health practitioners to attend appointments, the car mechanic to get your car serviced, or perhaps the library to take your books back on time. Your vet might even send messages to remind you to treat your pet with worming and flea prevention medication!

If you search an app store or the internet, you will quickly find a whole range of memory-related apps that provide calendars, alarms, notes, to-do lists, spaced recall timing schedules, organising ideas, reminder text messages and stress management! The resources list at the end of this book has some websites to get you started on your memory-app search.

Have you noticed that household appliances are becoming increasingly kind to us in terms of memory? Many electrical appliances, such as kettles and irons, now have built-in shut-off devices in case we forget to turn them off. Microwave ovens beep if we forget to take something out after we have cooked it, and the washing machine 'talks' to us when the washing is finished. We can attach automated timers to water taps and lights to turn them on and off. And that's just the beginning! Many people enjoy turning their houses into 'smart houses' run by automated systems or devices that respond to voice commands.

If you prefer a less technological approach, you can simply use an oven timer or inexpensive portable timer as a very handy household reminder device. You can set it to remind you to do many things—to turn the sprinkler off, to take the hand-washing out of the basin, or to wash the dye out of your hair. You just have to make sure you can hear the timer.

Where something is located

We can use location tracking technology to help us find many of our frequently lost possessions. A tracking device can be stuck to your keys, wallet, television remote control, and anything else that tends to go walkabout. These devices are readily available at electronics supply shops or online. When you lose an object that has a tracking tag stuck to it, you simply use an app on your phone to make the object sound an alarm. Some apps show you on a map where the object is located. You can also set up these systems so that they sound an alarm when the object is a certain distance from you.

Trevor had been working as a plumber for many years before he was involved in a car accident and suffered a head injury that left him with memory difficulties. When he returned to work, he found that he kept leaving his equipment at the houses he visited. He would get in his car after finishing a job, drive off, get to the next job, and realise that he couldn't do the job as he had left a vital tool at his previous job. These tools were often worth a lot of money, and he had already lost a few. I suggested that he put location tracking devices on his equipment—especially the expensive tools. That way he could program the tracking device to alert him when the specific tool was a certain distance away from him, and he could go back and get it straight away.

Anne

Many of us rely heavily on our smartphones these days to help manage our daily affairs, but they can be easily misplaced. It is so important to be able to find our smartphones, containing all our memory-support apps, that our phones often contain their own tracking device app.

I'd been on the go all day. I'd done the shopping, come home to unpack the shopping, taken our dog to the vet, come home again and then driven to my parents' house to take Dad to a doctor's appointment. When I finally got home again that night, I went to call a friend and couldn't find my phone. I panicked—it could be anywhere! I could have dropped it in the supermarket, at the vet's, at the doctor's. How was I going to find it? My daughter came to my rescue. 'Mum, all you need to do is use this app and it will show you where your phone is.' In just a few minutes, we had tracked my phone—I must have dropped it on the road when getting our dog out of the car. I often despair about what I see as negative effects of technology on our lives, but that phone tracking app is a definite positive!

Ming-zhu, 52

There have been some interesting innovations for frequently lost objects. You can buy an umbrella that not only sends an alert to your phone if you walk off without it, but also tells you whether you will need to take it according to the weather forecast! For those of us who repeatedly lose our glasses, you can now buy glasses with a tracking device built into them!

Of course, there are also phone apps to tell us where we parked our car, or you could simply use the camera in your phone to take a photo of where it is parked before you leave it. Many cars now have a built-in GPS (global positioning system) to assist us with remembering how to get to a particular location, or we can use a phone app to provide directions when we are driving, walking or using public transport.

Ask someone to remind you

People are often excellent external memory aids (or aides)! You can always ask someone to remind you.

Whenever we go away on holidays, I hide my jewellery in a special spot in the house. When we returned home from our last trip, it took me weeks to finally remember where I had hidden it! This year I am going to show my sister where it is hidden, so that she can remind me on our return.
Esme, 74

Other people also make willing external memory aides when it comes to recalling names. Don't be embarrassed to ask—many people experience difficulty with remembering from time to time. At a social gathering or meeting, you can quietly ask someone the name of a person that you are about to talk to, before you walk over to them. Alternatively, if you meet someone and you recognise their face but can't recall their name, it's okay to say, 'I recognise your face, but I can't recall your name at the moment.' You can sometimes even manage to have a conversation with someone without having to address them by their name.

I'm good at remembering faces, but not names. My wife is good at remembering names, but not faces. So whenever one of us has trouble recalling a name or a face, we just ask each other for help. We make a good pair!
Barry, 84

When we go to social gatherings, my husband helps with my poor memory for names. For example, if we walked up to a man called Greg, he would

include the name Greg at the start of our conversation, so that I could hear it. 'Hello, Greg, we haven't seen you for a while.'
Beth, 72

Rose works at a Senior Citizen's centre and has to greet dozens of people every day. She is 78 and has difficulty remembering their names. This is where her friend Joan comes in! Joan knows everyone's names. When someone comes up to Rose at the front desk, she says, 'Hello dear, how are you today?' Joan works in the kitchen behind the desk and when she hears Rose say, 'Hello dear', she comes up to the desk and immediately greets the person by name: 'Oh, Ian, nice to see you.' Rose can then also greet Ian, using his name. That's creative memory teamwork at its best!
Anne

Should I use internal or external memory strategies?

People sometimes think that it is 'lazy' to rely heavily on external strategies such as diaries, and may be concerned that it will make their memory worse: that they need to 'use it or lose it'. Drilling your memory, by repeating the same thing over and over in order to get it into your memory files, may help you to remember what you have been repeating, but it will not necessarily make your general memory abilities better. For example, with extensive repetition you might be able to remember a long shopping list 'in your head', but this doesn't mean that you will be any better at finding your car keys—and if you can't drive to the supermarket, then your memory of the shopping items will not be required!

> To reject memory aids when they could make life easier is like rejecting reading glasses when you need them . . . don't feel ashamed . . . what matters is that you continue to deal effectively with the environment.[1]

As we get older, we tend to favour external memory strategies over internal.[2] They are often easier to use; they can also be great fun and involve a bit of creativity, whereas the more complex internal strategies are not so 'user-friendly', requiring more time and a great deal of training and practice to master. Research shows that people tend to stop using complex internal strategies after a while. For instance, four months after a group of people had been trained to use the 'peg-word' method, half the people used it 'very little', and the other half did not use it at all.[3] Some memory researchers even make the confession that they do not use their own techniques when they leave the lab.

Everyday memory typically involves remembering things that we have seen or heard only once, or remembering to do something. For this type of daily memory use, external strategies are often more suitable. Researchers have found that external aids, including diaries and electronic reminder systems, are useful for remembering to do something.[4]

The way we live our lives these days can lead to information overload. There is so much to remember! Sometimes it is just not practical to try to remember all of this information using internal strategies alone. It makes good sense, then, to offload some of this information to back-up systems, that we can refer to should the need arise.

Using external strategies as back-up systems for remembering the more mundane aspects of life also leaves the mind more available for fun and creative pursuits. Instead of using up mental resources worrying about what needs to be remembered, you can turn your often limited attention elsewhere, and perhaps discover new things. For example, you can fill your diary up with names and appointments, and in your memory filing cabinet reserve your energy and time for organising the storage of more exciting information. This way, you will be able to more efficiently sort through your memories when you want to recall information.

Albert Einstein is often quoted as an example of this approach. Apparently he said that he wouldn't waste his mental energy on memorising his home phone number because it would only take a minute to look this information up. Einstein had other, more exciting, ideas that he wanted to occupy his mind with.

Using the strategies that suit you best

I interviewed a 73-year-old man at the kitchen table in his derelict house hundreds of kilometres from Melbourne. The first time I asked him when a particular event occurred, he stopped, then silently rose to a standing position and walked to the outside door; he stood there, peered outside and returned to his seat and answered '1956'. About two minutes later I asked another question, about his family. Again he rose, walked outside, went to the doorway and peered out, and when he returned sat down and proudly said '8th May 1961'. It just didn't make sense, so I asked, 'What takes you to the door?' He answered—with a glint in his eyes—'All my important dates are painted on my outside water tank and the one way to remember them is to get up and look.'
Julie, 52

When it comes down to it, the best memory strategies for you, as an individual, are the ones that you prefer, and the ones that work best for your own unique situation. You will probably use a mixture of internal and external strategies that suit you and your lifestyle.

The strategies that you use now will also depend on what strategies you have used for memory management in the past. We tend to stick to what we are familiar with. You may also notice that your need for, and use of, strategies fluctuates over time. When we are busy, and our workload is heavy, it can be useful to rely more on external strategies, which use less of our available mental energy.

I used to try to keep all my 'to do' plans in my head, but now things have changed. I'm a lot busier—in a managerial role at work. I'm now in my mid-thirties, and I can't rely on 'my head' to remind me, because if I forget something important at work, I'm in trouble! I've noticed that I have begun to write 'to do' lists on scraps of paper, which I carry around everywhere with me. The only problem with this is that sometimes I can't find the piece of paper. The other day I left it in a meeting, and when I eventually remembered where I had left it, and went back to collect it, someone told me that they had thrown it out.

Gene, 36

Gene obviously finds that having a written memory back-up system gives him peace of mind. To make it work even better for him, he might find it useful to write his 'to do' list in his phone or appointment diary at work, and get into the habit of checking his list regularly. This way he will avoid losing the list, and always remember to look at it because it has become part of his daily routine.

As you have been reading about the many different memory strategies, you most likely have found some that are very familiar, some new ones that appeal to you and others that you could never imagine using. You may also use some that have not been mentioned. Tell someone about these and check if they also use some strategies that are not described here. Talking about memory strategies reinforces the fact that they are as important as any other area of our own self-care, and this will contribute in turn to our developing more 'memory-wise' communities.

I listened to a great radio talk-back session on diaries. People were calling in and talking about the types of diaries that they preferred to use. The callers were quite passionate about their diaries. One woman said she buys the same paper diary every year, and will never change. One man said he had given up on his digital diary because he likes to be able to see the whole week ahead, and to visualise this in his head. Other people said they could never go back to paper diaries, as they don't have a 'search' button and they don't provide text reminders to their phones to tell them to do something. There were some interesting suggestions for combining paper and digital strategies. One woman said that she takes a photo of her paper diary with her phone so that she has a copy with her when she is out and about.

Anne

Everyone is different, and we all have our own preferences for memory strategies. For example, some people find that visual strategies suit them best, while others find that they need to write things down in words if they are to be any use later.

Whenever Rana gives me directions, I have a lot of difficulty following them. She likes to describe the route we are to travel in words, telling me about certain features along the way that I will see as I drive past. I much prefer a picture to guide me—an actual map I can see, and then visualise in my memory as I drive.

Chloe, 65

The type of strategy you use will also depend on your lifestyle and personal interests. What do you need to remember? Are you trying to find your wallet? Are you trying to recall someone's name? Where are you at the time? Are you driving a car, and not able to write something down? You will probably have found that you need to use a different strategy for each situation.

No one can tell you which memory strategies will work best for you as an individual. Managing your memory is a dynamic and personal process, and may change substantially over your lifetime. General guidelines may be helpful, but even these can only be applied to the extent that they suit your lifestyle. *Strategies need to suit you so that you will actually use them.*

What is important is that you are aware that there are strategies you can draw on to get the most out of your memory. You will probably find you already have a range of particular strategies for specific situations that you encounter. It may be useful to review your current needs, and decide whether you need to 'polish up' your strategies, or develop new ones. Be creative!

Key points

- Memory strategies can enhance everyday memory and make you feel more confident that you will remember to remember.
- You don't need to remember everything!
- Tell yourself to 'stay calm' because panic will only make remembering more difficult.
- Pay attention to paying attention!
- Use organisation and routine to support memory.
- When you think you need to remember something, do it now, 'or do something now to help you remember to do it later.
- Use a combination of internal (mental) and external (memory aids) strategies.
- Strategies need to suit you so that you will use them—choose the ones that work best for you.
- As life circumstances change, there may be benefits in testing out new memory strategies.

CHAPTER 7

Working and learning

Not so long ago, people tended to stay in the same job for most of their working lives and retire from that same job. Not anymore! Careers these days usually involve frequent job changes, which means we are dealing with constant change in our workplaces. We are consistently trying to make the unfamiliar more familiar: a new job, a new role, new co-workers, perhaps new technology, or even working in a different country. All this change means an increased load on everybody's memories—for the old and the young.

If you are one of the few who does stay with the same company and in the same job for many years, you will see the job itself change, as new technology permeates the workplace. Information technology requires constant updating of knowledge, which is much easier for younger workers who have grown up with it. Older workers may require regular training to maintain familiarity and confidence with the technology which seems second nature to younger staffers.

Demands for increased quality and tougher competition force all of us to continually upgrade our skills. We are constantly pushed to learn, improve and adapt. Apart from our own specific work skills, we are now required to learn things not directly related to our job—like emergency procedures, and occupational health and safety protocols.

Often it's a matter of 'too much to do in too little time'. It's easy to become overwhelmed with juggling information, decisions and things to do. We may have too many distractions, too much inform-ation and too many choices. We are often deluged with incoming information—texts, phone calls, emails, social media alerts, and still some paper-based mail and information—which we shift to another spot, waiting for the time to respond to or sort through. Unexpected demands are placed on us: we might be requested to prepare a report at the last minute or do the job of two people. A huge volume of work causes anxiety or stress, which often leads to further strain on our ability to remember.

Being an older person at work

We are likely to work to an older age than our parents' generation. Many people in their fifties or sixties may be happy to retire from full-time work, but still want to remain useful and active. Some seek part-time employment, others may start their own small busi-ness. Many want to take up skills and learning opportunities they didn't have time for before. Older adults may return to study, work from home, work part time, or do voluntary work. They may have to juggle more than one work responsibility, and there may often be family responsibilities too.

'Old' is very relative. Being over 40 may be considered 'over the hill' in some younger workforces, but in others you're not considered to be getting older until you are over 65. We might be five or ten or twenty years older than others at work, which may be viewed by ourselves as being senior, more experienced. But not everybody may see it that way; often being older can be seen as a disadvantage, sometimes even by ourselves.

Some people feel at the height of their powers as an older adult, with a world of experience to guide them soundly. Others feel squeezed out of work roles on the grounds of age, or when re-entering the workplace face implicit discrimination, sometimes among fellow staff as well as management. Self-consciousness because of age can have a negative impact on work performance. Pride in experience helps to counteract this concern.

I felt really happy to turn 50, so I gave myself a birthday party at work. Never again! After this I was never just Kate, I was Kate who is 50 and 'different', and I felt discriminated against because of my age for the first time.
Kate, 50

Older people may experience some mild changes in their memory processes. They may find concentration and attention less acute, and that it takes longer to retrieve names and events from memory storage (as described in Chapter 2)—but strengths in procedural memories (how to do things) and the wisdom of experience usually outweigh these relative inefficiencies. Using strategies to compensate can help to boost confidence.

Be aware of distractions

Being more susceptible to distraction is often a frustration for older people. It shows up when you're doing more than one thing at a time, or when your attention is being called for by several things at once. It can be hard to ignore distractions, switch between tasks or pick up where you left off. At work, we are increasingly required to do several things at once—like waiting 'on hold' on the phone while maybe simultaneously reading documents or checking emails, so as not to waste time.

The workplace has many potential distractions, especially in open-plan offices and staff common rooms, where co-workers often can't find their volume knobs! Common distractions might come from noise, people talking, alerts sounding on your phone or computer, radio or music playing, buzzing flies, flapping blinds or building works outside your window.

There are always people talking in my shared office. If I really need to concentrate on something, I move somewhere else.
Kay, 42

Our office clown had this annoying habit of walking around in fits of laughter, making jokes whenever he felt like it. Finally I plucked up the courage to assert myself and told him how distracting I found it.
Andrea, 46

Distractions at work throw me off now. I'll start doing something, like writing an email, and get distracted and go on to doing something else. Ages later I realise that I didn't send the email that I had been working on before.
Dee, 58

I'll be in the middle of fitting a tap and my phone will ring. I want to answer it, but I know I'm likely to forget what the person is saying because I'm distracted. I've worked out it's better not to answer the call when I'm in the middle of a job. I return all my calls later in the day, when I can pay full attention to what the person is saying, and jot down any important details.
Ted, 56

We can also be distracted by things we see—people moving in our line of sight, changing lighting, messages coming up on our screens, and clutter. Clutter may be documents, notes, client files or receipts all in a jumble on your computer desktop or your actual desk. It could be unsorted stuff in your drawers or your files. Maybe it is the 67 new email messages in your inbox when you log on to the computer! This external clutter affects our ability to concentrate, and makes it harder to remember where we have put things. It can be distracting and harder to focus, so the aim is to keep it out of sight.

To '**de-clutter**', it helps to:

- screen information as soon as it arrives
- throw out what you don't need to read or keep (ask yourself, 'Will I really use it?')
- check emails less frequently, and decide whether you really need to be on so many copy lists.

I found if I changed the position of my computer, I was less distracted by seeing people walking past me.
Stuart, 56

Our own thoughts and concerns can also be distracting. You might be distracted by your emotions if you have just returned to work after a disturbing event. You might be a carer, concerned about the needs of a person left at home. Parents at work can often feel a sense of guilt and anxiety about leaving their children in someone else's care. A colleague at work might be standing over you, making you anxious. You might be in a state of panic because you are running late for an important appointment or job interview. You can also experience stress from highly significant events—you can be just as distracted by an exciting surprise as by something awful.

If we are not able to pay attention, then we can't expect to get the most out of our abilities to remember. To improve your likelihood of paying attention, think about:

- arriving ahead of time for appointments and meetings, and spending the extra time preparing for the meeting
- avoiding over-scheduling, which makes it impossible to be on time, and easy to succumb to stress, worry and fatigue
- deferring any new learning situation, or making sure it can be repeated soon, if you are really tired from not sleeping well
- building time into your life for emotional emergencies, physical activity and fun!
- planning for 10 minutes a day of mental space, or meditation, or being in a quiet place—even lying in the bath thinking of nothing at all.

Focus on just one thing at a time whenever possible, and work on ways to reduce possible distractions that can make you irritable, anxious and affect your ability to remember at work. A quiet, organised workplace is an asset at any age but, as we get older, may become more of a necessity.

See Chapter 3 for other factors that could be adversely affecting your work performance, and Chapter 6 for more ideas on enhancing attention.

Learning new tricks

No matter what age we are, we do not stop learning. Our workplaces demand that we regularly learn new things and update our knowledge. We might be offered training courses, asked to read instruction manuals, or attend seminars to learn new information. It seems that there is always new technology to master—a new smartphone, new computer software system, or new television with a complicated remote-control device. Many older people engage in voluntary work, and also like to develop hobbies, interests or intellectual opportunities. There are courses for anything and everything—ballroom dancing, watercolour painting, or even training your dog! A new job, technological device or hobby might be enticing, but can lead to anxiety, with a feeling of, 'I'm too old for that.' As we get older, we sometimes doubt our ability to learn new things. This makes sense: the research into ageing tells us that it may take longer to learn new things because we are often slower to encode and retrieve new information from memory storage than we were in our younger years.

The important news is that we all can, and do, learn new things, no matter what age we are. We just need to accept that this process may take more time as we age, and be harder to master. All we need to do is adapt our learning by being strategic!

If I do something myself, I remember; if someone shows me, I don't.
Vera, 62

'I hear and I forget, I see and I remember, I do and I understand'
is an old saying that captures well how we learn. When learning
something new in a group setting such as a **seminar**, become as
actively involved as possible:

- Process the information in as many ways as possible—examine
  any visual aids, take notes and draw diagrams.
- Ask questions and join in discussions.
- Volunteer to participate in demonstrations or activities, and go
  over the key points on your way home.
- If possible, run through the points you want to recall with a
  friend or colleague the next day.

A **training course** generally offers opportunities to practise
newly learned skills:

- Watch any demonstrations carefully and ask questions. The
  more you understand the new information, the easier it will be
  to remember it later.
- Actively practise each step of the task yourself.
- If you make mistakes, don't be overly concerned; mistakes are
  an important part of learning.
- Keep personalised notes next to any equipment that you are
  learning how to use.
- Finding a sympathetic tutor is a great help, and younger ones
  can help imbue enthusiasm and confidence; just make sure they
  work at your pace! Ask the person who is teaching you to go
  slowly, and to repeat themselves if necessary.
- Practise the new skill straight after you have been shown how to
  do it, following the notes that you have written down. Use 'spaced
  recall' to consolidate the information. Do this by practising the

new skill repeatedly, but slowly increasing the length of time between practice.

When learning from **reading books**, processing the information at a deeper level helps to anchor information in your memory. You can do this by:

- highlighting important information
- making notes in the margin
- drawing diagrams of new information
- writing summaries of the key new concepts or information in your own words, or reading the information out loud to yourself
- linking the information to other related information that you already know well
- quizzing yourself about the information at increasing time intervals after reading it
- teaching someone else the new information, which is a great way to consolidate your learning.

When **learning instructions** for how to use a new piece of equipment, it can help if you:

- Actively try out each step as you read it in the instruction manual, and even talk out loud as you practise each new step.
- Write out in your own words, or draw a diagram of, the steps required to operate the piece of equipment.
- Check online for video instructions for the appliance.
- Go to the shop you bought the appliance or device from, and ask them to show you how to use it.
- Put personalised step-by-step instructions on, or next to, new equipment, devices or appliances, so you can follow your instructions again the next time you use them.

We can learn new things at any age; it's just a matter of being realistic and creative in the ways we do it. Think positive and challenge yourself to learn something new. Learn the information as actively as possible, and practise recalling the information at increasing time intervals. Once you have succeeded with learning something new, you might feel so good about your learning potential that you decide to teach someone else some new tricks!

Memory strategies at work

Sometimes it's not until you change jobs that you realise there were many structures that provided memory cues in your old workplace that you had taken for granted. Perhaps there were noticeboards in the staffroom, or 'in/out boards' telling you when to expect your colleagues back at the office. You might have been supplied with schedules for regular meetings at the beginning of the year. Such routines and cues lessen the load on memory. When they are changed, or not practised or promoted in the new workplace, it is easy to feel all at sea. You will continue to be distracted for a couple of weeks, until you are reoriented and comfortably familiar with your new environment.

Having an organised system and a degree of routine and regularity in the workplace allows us to feel in control. It is a relief to be able to locate items you need the first time you look for them. It lessens anxiety and promotes self-confidence. We end up having more time to be creative because we spend less time searching. Of course, there is no single, perfect way to organise your workplace; it depends on your job and the way you like to do things.

Organised storage: putting things in special places

We discussed the benefits of storing things in special places in Chapter 6. Having designated locations for work-related objects makes it easier to recall where they are kept. You could store your spare paper and ink next to the printer, or your tools in your van ready for the next service call. Store the objects you use most often close to hand, and those used less often, further away. If you store items in boxes, use clear plastic containers so you can see what is in them. Colour coding can help and labelling is essential so that others will know where you have stored things too. Always make sure that you return items to their special place!

I travel regularly for my work, so I make sure I always have a jacket on that has two pockets inside it. In one pocket I put my passport and plane ticket, and in the other I put my mobile phone and wallet. This routine allows me not to have to worry about these little things, because I know they are always there. I'd be lost without this system—I even had to wear my jacket yesterday when it was 38 degrees!
Peter, 42

Filing

It had to happen soon—the piles on my desk were like volcanoes ready to erupt. In fact, one pile had erupted regularly over the last few months. With a slight nudge, the pile of papers had fallen all over the desk more than once. I had so much paperwork for various projects that I had made piles all over the floor. Only trouble was that I kept forgetting which pile was which, and I couldn't find particular bits of information that I knew were there, but I just couldn't locate! Finally, I decided enough was enough. I gave my office a storage makeover. I bought some new shelves, storage boxes and folders. I created labelled spots for each project on my new shelves. I created folders for all those loose bits of paper that I had collected and slowly got rid of those volcano piles on my desk. I threw out a whole box of papers that I didn't need anymore. My memory feels like it has improved, but really all I have done is organised a small part of my life.
Ralph, 62

If you have an organised digital and/or paper-based filing system, you don't need to rely on your memory of where files are stored. If you are not at work, your colleagues should be able to locate files in your absence. An efficient filing system has:

- clear labels that will make it easier for you and for others to find and use these resources
- files that are regularly 'de-cluttered', containing only significant and up-to-date items
- colour coding, if possible, for ready identification.

Ideas for categorising your files include:

- personal file—e.g. personal correspondence, résumé, performance evaluation
- current project files—e.g. courses you are attending, projects
- operational files—e.g. budget, accounts, staff meetings, newsletters
- equipment instructions file
- forms file—e.g. tax form, invoice form.

On your desk

It would be unrealistic to expect that our desks will be spotless at all times. The aim is to have a clear workspace and be able to find things when we need them. Some of the most obvious ways to keep order bear repeating, though. An in-tray where you can put newly arrived materials in preparation for sorting, an out-tray for completed items prior to distribution, and a pending tray for non-urgent items, together with a 'to do' list, will greatly simplify the load for your memory.

Every day at work I get phone calls on different topics, which leads to more piles of messages recorded on paper, which seem to cover more and more desk space. I've found it much easier to locate the messages I'm looking for after I grabbed a batch of folders and cleared the pile up.
Simon, 48

'Pick-up' points

It is very frustrating to arrive at work and realise that you have left the tool you need for the job in your garage, or your report at home on the dining-room table. Creating pick-up points at home and at work can help with remembering to take something from home into work, or vice versa. Many people use their work bag as a pick-up point, or a table by the door you exit from. Put what you need at the pick-up point as soon as you think of it. Get into the habit of always checking this spot as you leave.

Half the week I'm based in Australia and the rest of the week I'm overseas. I've learned from experience that I need to take half an hour or so, before I leave, to run through in my mind each meeting that I will be going to, and what I will need to take with me to each. I do this because I'm terrified of being an idiot in a meeting because I have forgotten to bring something.
Sharon, 53

I keep a digital copy of all my files in an online file-sharing application, so that I can work on a file at any of my work sites.
Nassim, 45

Maintaining good organisation

All these ideas sound good in theory, but in practice they can be hard to maintain, especially if you are sharing an office or workspace.

Joe doesn't think he is messy, but he is. I can never see any bench space, and it drives me mad. Twice a year I clean out all the files and put them in order, but he thinks it's a waste of time.
Rita, 54, Joe's wife

You will only continue to use a system that suits you as an individual, so set it up in a way you like, that fits your needs at work. Some people like clean surfaces; others work quite happily with their work space covered with objects. Build a regular 10–15 minute time slot into the end of your day to clear the top of your desk, or if you are not in the office each day, it might suit you better to do this once a week.

Writing things down

Writing things down is the most common technique used to help us remember things, as discussed in Chapter 6. At work, a paper or digital diary is an important written memory aid in which you can note down important information to remember. Keep your diary system streamlined—don't be tempted to write reminders in too many different locations, otherwise you will waste time trying to recall where you wrote that important note!

A few weeks ago, a friend in my team told me about a new place to buy some equipment for work. I typed the name and address of the warehouse into my phone, but now I can't find where I typed it, and I want to go there today. My phone is full of random notes and reminders in different apps! I'm going to have to work out a simpler system so I can get my hands on information when I need it.
Maani, 63

A digital diary can be programmed to provide timely reminders. If you prefer to use a paper-based diary, leave it somewhere you will see it often, and check it regularly for appointments, meetings and project deadlines. Put reminders in on the appropriate days. For example, if you are presenting some information at a particular meeting, write a note in well before this date to remind you to start preparing what you will present. A secondary wall calendar or yearly planner can be helpful for remembering future projects and planning for their deadlines.

I have several projects on the go, which I used to manage in my head, and I often couldn't remember which job needed to be done first. Now I write them in my diary in order of importance. I find I can devote more time to my work, rather than trying to remember what to do next.
Anna, 56

A 'to do' list helps you remember things that you need or would like to do that day, or even in the next few days, such as returning a phone call, writing an email or preparing the agenda for a meeting. Of course, it is not a list of *everything* you do each day, as this would be far too long—but it acts as a reminder of things that you may *forget* to do, and it helps with prioritising your jobs. Keep your 'to do' list somewhere you frequently see it, for quick reference. Digital 'to do' lists can be programmed to provide reminders at specified times. You can ask a colleague or friend to assist with maintaining your 'to do' list, and to run through the list with you on a regular basis.

I have an A4-sized diary with a page to a day. I jot down my daily tasks into my diary and cross them out when I have done them. At the end of each day I write the things that I didn't get done onto the next page.
Tony, 39

A memory-wise work environment

Constant change in our workplaces, and an increasing proportion of older workers, means that we need to actively promote more memory-wise work and learning environments. Practical changes should be introduced to reduce the demand on memory and to maximise the likelihood that new information can be learned. Workplaces need to acknowledge memory problems. If it is not okay to talk about memory difficulties, this can lead to anxiety, which in turn can exacerbate any memory problems.

A memory-wise workplace does the following:

- simplifies work processes and work instructions
- arranges for work instructions to be available in written and verbal formats
- highlights and repeats important information

- avoids information overload
- allows time for questions, clarification and practice
- gives permission for people to be reminded
- creatively uses aids to reinforce memory, particularly visual aids
- controls noise and other distractions
- encourages people to disclose memory concerns.

Challenge your workplace: how seriously does it take being memory-wise?

We have a high turnover of casual staff at my work, and it has been difficult to remember all of their names. A bright spark at work came up with a great solution to this problem. All staff now have their name, role and photo displayed on the work intranet, arranged by departments. I don't know why we hadn't done this earlier—it has made such a difference!
Vanda, 66

Key points   WORKING AND LEARNING

- Constant changes in our workplaces mean an increased load on everybody's memories, no matter what age we are.
- Older people at work may need to use strategies to compensate for mild changes in their memory abilities.
- Being more susceptible to distraction is often a frustration for older people, and working on ways to reduce possible distractions becomes a necessity.
- We can learn new things at any age if we adapt our learning by being strategic.
- Having an organised system and a degree of routine and regularity in the workplace allows us to feel in control.
- We need to promote more memory-wise work and learning environments.

CHAPTER 8

What if it's dementia?

When I went to visit Audrey, a 72-year-old woman, her geriatrician had just told her that she had dementia. Together with her husband Tom, we talked about what this news meant to them as a couple. Tom said that on the way home from the appointment with the geriatrician, he had said to Audrey, 'Today is just another day; we are no different from yesterday, we just have different knowledge from yesterday.'

Anne

Tom's words reminded me of a past catch-cry of our local dementia support organisation: 'Life doesn't stop when dementia starts.' Indeed, life doesn't stop with a diagnosis of dementia—there is plenty more living to do. This chapter provides information about dementia—what it is, how it is diagnosed, and the latest on medical treatment. Being memory-wise when you have dementia involves looking after your psychological and physical health, as well as supporting your memory with practical memory strategies.

What is dementia?

One way to think about dementia is to see it as evidence of a progressive change of brain functioning. Dementia is an illness that can cause memory loss, together with decline in other areas of thinking ability and emotional processing. These changes impact upon your ability to function in everyday life. We hear many words used to describe the existence of progressive memory loss, which can be confusing. Terms you might have heard are 'dementia', 'Alzheimer's disease' and 'vascular dementia'.

The brain change involved in dementia can have many different causes, just as a high temperature is a sign of body change that could stem from a variety of illnesses. There are several causes of dementia, and the most common is 'Alzheimer's disease'. Up to 70 per cent of all cases of dementia involve Alzheimer's disease. So, when we say the words 'Alzheimer's disease' and 'dementia', we often mean the same thing.

What causes dementia apart from Alzheimer's disease?

Vascular dementia is the next most common cause of dementia, accounting for approximately 15–20 per cent of dementia cases. It arises from problems with the circulation of blood to the brain. Vascular dementia is typically caused by a succession of minor strokes, which people often aren't aware of having, and changes in memory, thinking abilities and emotional processing can occur. Many people with dementia have a mixture of both Alzheimer's disease and vascular dementia. In a much smaller number of cases, dementia may be related to other conditions, such as fronto-temporal dementia, dementia with Lewy bodies, Parkinson's disease, Huntington's disease, long-term alcoholism, HIV/AIDS and rare degenerative diseases of the brain.

This chapter will concentrate on Alzheimer's disease because this is the most common cause of dementia, and the focus of much anxiety in people concerned about memory loss.

What causes Alzheimer's disease?

The symptoms of Alzheimer's disease are caused by brain cells becoming disconnected, malfunctioning and ultimately dying. Scientists are becoming increasingly sure that this is at least in part due to the presence of an abnormal toxic protein, known as amyloid, which accumulates in the brain.

Scientists still don't really understand why some people develop Alzheimer's disease and some don't. It is likely due to a combination of inherited genetic risk factors interacting with non-genetic factors. This is similar to the way in which inherited factors make some people more likely to get heart disease or breast cancer than others.

Having a close relative with the disease, such as a parent, is seen as an inherited risk factor, and may increase your chances of getting Alzheimer's disease by a small amount—but it doesn't mean you are destined to develop it. In a small number of cases, Alzheimer's disease occurs because of a genetic mutation (that is, the illness is inherited from an affected parent). This rare inherited form of early-onset Alzheimer's disease ('autosomal-dominant Alzheimer's disease') accounts for around 1 per cent of all people with dementia, and typically develops when people are in their forties or fifties.[1]

Researchers have identified several health and lifestyle risk factors that may make Alzheimer's disease a little more likely for some people. Risk factors at midlife include high blood pressure, obesity and hearing loss, and risk factors during later life include diabetes, smoking, depression, physical inactivity and social isolation. By contrast, a protective factor identified is spending more time in education during childhood.[2] (For more information about reducing the risk of developing dementia, see Chapter 5.)

At what age are you most likely to develop Alzheimer's disease?

The proportion of people developing Alzheimer's disease increases with age, but the majority of older people *do not* develop the disease before their lives end. Approximately 3 per cent of people aged 70–74 develop dementia, as compared to 18 per cent of people aged 85–89.[3] Women are more likely than men to develop dementia in their lifetimes. One reason for this is that more women live to an advanced age than men, and new research is investigating the role of certain hormones in the development and progression of Alzheimer's disease.[4]

How is dementia diagnosed?

There are many different pathways towards an assessment for possible dementia. The most usual procedure (it will vary from state to state, country to country) involves consultation with your doctor, who may then refer you to a specialist in the diagnosis and management of memory and thinking problems. Such specialists include geriatricians, psychiatrists, neuropsychologists and neurologists.

Other conditions that can cause changes in memory functioning include anxiety, depression, stroke, tumours, vitamin deficiencies, infections, thyroid disease and many other illnesses. Investigations performed to check for these include a clinical examination, blood tests, and brain scans such as CT (computerised tomography) or MRI (magnetic resonance imaging). Doctors will sometimes arrange more specialised brain scans, such as SPECT (single-photon emission computerised tomography) and PET (positron emission tomography), or amyloid PET imaging (usually through clinical research trials).

Correct diagnosis of the cause of dementia is important because management, prognosis and potential inheritability of different conditions vary widely.

What is involved in memory assessment or testing?

In Australia, memory specialists can be consulted privately or through a memory clinic. A typical memory clinic has a team which may include geriatricians, psychiatrists, neurologists, nurses, neuropsychologists, speech pathologists, occupational therapists and social workers. People are usually referred to the clinic by their regular doctor. The person who is thought to have memory difficulties is seen by one of the doctors in the clinic, and the person's family is interviewed by a team member to gather information about how and when the memory problem developed. This stage is important because when people have memory difficulties, they are often not able to give exact details concerning the nature and extent of their own problem. The memory clinic team conducts a detailed assessment and provides feedback to the person who has had their memory assessed, together with family members. Follow-up appointments can be scheduled to monitor progress and to discuss ongoing management.

As well as a physical examination, an assessment of memory and other thinking abilities is performed. This can vary from simple tests to a more detailed neuropsychological assessment. A doctor will often use brief tests of memory and thinking, which are useful because they are quick and easy to use, and interpreting them does not require extensive training. However, they do not always pick up mild or subtle memory difficulties—and, if they do, they may not provide enough information to assist with finding the cause of the memory problem. Nor do these brief tests examine a person's abilities in enough detail to be helpful with planning for future care. Sometimes a doctor will refer onwards for more comprehensive assessment of memory and thinking abilities—by a neuropsychologist, for instance.

How is Alzheimer's disease different from normal memory loss?

Everyday memory problems can be frustrating, but they don't pose a threat to your ability to function independently. Normal everyday memory lapses are often the result of not paying close attention. We might notice that we can still learn something new if we are interested enough, and make an effort to do so. Memory can play more tricks on us as we get older when we are out of routine (see Chapter 2), or when we are experiencing changes in our health or lifestyle, as described in Chapters 3 and 4.

If you have Alzheimer's disease, you may require assistance with everyday activities you used to do independently. You might forget how to do things that you have always been very good at—such as how to cook a meal that you have made regularly in the past, or how to use the washing machine that you have had for years. It could be difficult for you to remember your home address, or you might become lost in familiar surroundings.

My wife has just been diagnosed with Alzheimer's disease. Over the past three years her memory has gradually gone from bad to worse. She always had a good memory, but now things just don't sink in—I answer her questions and she asks me the same thing again straight away. She forgets where things are kept around the house and keeps putting them in new locations, and of course can't find them later. She has been lost on several occasions in shopping centres.

Now her memory for the past is slipping, too. The other day someone asked her what her job was when she was younger, and she couldn't tell them. I've also noticed that she puts on the same clothes day after day. She used to be so meticulous about her appearance. Thank goodness she can still enjoy her music and the grandchildren—it's nice to see her enjoying herself.

Chris, 82

Mild cognitive impairment

After a medical assessment of memory, some people are told that they have 'mild cognitive impairment'. This term is used when people have memory loss that is more than expected with the ageing process, but not severe enough to warrant a diagnosis of dementia. When people have mild cognitive impairment, they experience regular and often frustrating memory lapses, but they can still carry out their everyday activities independently. Doctors usually recommend medical review after one to two years because in people diagnosed with mild cognitive impairment, there is an increased risk of developing dementia due to Alzheimer's disease. The underlying disease process of Alzheimer's disease is thought to build up over many years before the memory loss becomes more obvious,[5] and for some people, 'mild cognitive impairment' reflects a very early stage in this disease process. Despite this risk, around one-third of people who are diagnosed as having mild cognitive impairment do not experience significant deterioration in their memory over time.

Can I tell if someone else has dementia?

This chapter has outlined some areas where the memory change of those with Alzheimer's disease is different from the problems of everyday memory functioning. This difference isn't always clear. Assessing whether memory change is part of normal ageing or a sign of early dementia can be one of the more difficult diagnostic challenges for memory specialists.

This book will certainly not provide enough information to allow people to work out whether they have Alzheimer's disease or not. Nor can a memory specialist make conclusions from single instances of memory loss. If someone says, 'My father repeats himself in the same conversation—do you think he has dementia?', it would not be possible to answer them with certainty. People with and without dementia repeat themselves in conversation. One would need to know more about how often it happens, under what circumstances, how long it has been happening, what other changes have accompanied it, and so on. A comprehensive physical and memory assessment might be the best course if it is of real concern for the person.

What medical treatments are available for Alzheimer's disease?

A great deal of the current research into Alzheimer's disease looks at potential medical treatments. Most studies focus on drugs designed to slow or halt the decline that characterises the illness. Stop-press announcements about possible new treatments for Alzheimer's disease hit the headlines from time to time. Most new discoveries require much investigation over many years before they can be transformed into procedures, medications or preventive behaviours. Medical science is 'evidence-based' and relies on studies and trials to work out whether treatments are helpful. When trying to assess the significance of new 'breakthroughs', give more weight to announcements that have been published in scientific journals subject to review by other scientists, and to those where the results have been repeated by more than one set of investigators.

Research and new developments are taking place all the time, so any information on medical treatments can quickly become outdated. It is important that you seek up-to-date specialist knowledge for your own situation.

The best current evidence for effective treatment of Alzheimer's disease is for drugs called cholinesterase inhibitors, which raise the level of a chemical called acetylcholine, which is essential for memory formation within the brain. Drugs of this type include donepezil (Aricept), rivastigmine (Exelon) and galantamine (Reminyl), and these medications all work in a similar way. In people with mild to moderate Alzheimer's disease, these medications may produce mild improvement in functioning, and there may not be the same degree of decline over the next few years as there would have been without the medication. It should be emphasised that any improvement is modest in most cases, and these medications have the potential to cause side-effects such as nausea, diarrhoea, vivid dreams, leg cramps and increased sweating. Side-effects prevent around one in eight people who are started on these drugs from continuing with them. A medication called memantine (Ebixa) is sometimes prescribed for people in the later stages of Alzheimer's disease. People with dementia are also sometimes prescribed additional medications if they experience symptoms of depression, anxiety or psychosis.

Scientists continue to investigate the possible benefits of nutritional supplements for people with Alzheimer's disease. There have been many studies examining the potential benefit of antioxidants, such as vitamin E and ginkgo biloba, but the potential benefit of antioxidants in Alzheimer's disease remains to be fully defined.[6]

More recently, scientists have examined the therapeutic potential of specific combinations of nutrients. 'Souvenaid' is a nutritional supplement containing a combination of nutrients that has been developed for people who have Alzheimer's disease. Souvenaid has been shown to enhance the membranes of brain cells and the synaptic connections between them, which is thought to help slow decline in memory and thinking abilities during dementia.[7]

A wide range of other drugs are under investigation for the treatment and prevention of Alzheimer's disease. Dementia support organisations (listed in the 'Resources' section at the end of this book) often distribute useful information about new treatments, and can refer people to specialists in the field who can provide expert advice and information about clinical research trials that you may wish to take part in.

Medical advice should be sought before taking any medication for Alzheimer's disease or its prevention, whether or not it is prescribed, or bought over the counter in a pharmacy or health food store, because of the possibility of harmful side-effects and negative outcomes of interactions between drugs.

With no medical cure available for Alzheimer's disease at present, management involves ensuring maximum quality of life for the person with dementia, and the provision of considerable support to families and carers.

What helps when the diagnosis is dementia?

If the diagnosis is dementia, it can be hard to know what to do next. It may be helpful finally to know what the problem is, and to understand why memory issues have been such a problem over recent times. Nonetheless, most people feel very emotional when being told about what the problems with memory are likely to be. It is normal to feel worried, anxious, angry, lonely or sad.

Be aware that the memory and thinking difficulties that you experience are happening because of a memory illness—don't blame yourself for these changes. Be patient and take time to work out new ways of coping. It is common to feel embarrassed about telling others or to find it difficult to share your feelings, or even to talk about your fears, but it can be helpful to talk to other people who are dealing with the challenges of memory loss. Your local dementia support organisation can put you in contact with others who have been diagnosed with dementia.

There are many things you can do to take more control over your situation, so you can remain as independent as possible and continue to enjoy life. For example, focusing on the things that you *can* do well is a good start to remaining positive. Looking closely at health and lifestyle issues can make a real difference. Practical strategies can help to increase confidence, reduce anxiety and get around the problems of memory loss. Making small changes can make a big difference.

People with dementia often ask, 'What can I do to improve my memory?' There is a lot you can do to maximise your memory function at any point in time. As explained in Chapter 3, our memory fluctuates for a variety of reasons, which is the same when you have dementia. The graph below, of memory change over time during dementia,[8] shows your maximum potential memory function as line A at the top. Underneath this line is a wiggly line B, representing your actual everyday memory function, which changes from day to day, moment to moment. Your memory loss can be worse when you are physically sick, feeling down, or dealing with something unfamiliar, like moving house. It's important to identify any health and lifestyle factors that may be exacerbating your memory difficulties, and work on ways to keep your everyday memory function as close to the line of maximum potential memory function as possible.

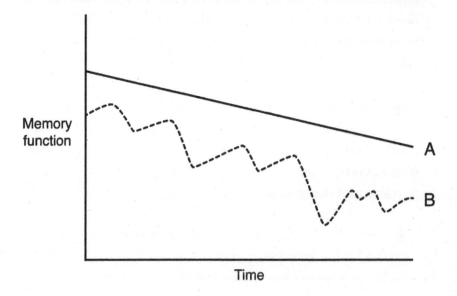

Health

We discussed how important good health is to memory in Chapter 3. Looking after your physical and mental health is important when you have a memory illness. Any health problems can make your memory difficulties worse, and it is important to seek medical help for these problems.

- **Illness, physical discomfort or pain**. Memory loss can worsen at times of significant pain, or with infections, such as urinary tract or chest infections. People sometimes notice acute confusion after general anaesthesia for surgery. Be aware that some of the fluctuations you notice in your memory could be related to other illnesses, which of course should be treated appropriately.
- Keeping healthy involves getting some sort of regular **physical activity**, such as walking or gardening; eating a **well-balanced diet**; regular rest and relaxation; and having a regular check-up with your doctor.
- Make sure you take any prescribed **medication** (tips to help with remembering to take medication will be described later in this chapter). Check with your doctor to see if any current medications may have a detrimental effect on memory.
- **Alcohol**. Dementia can make you more sensitive to the effects of alcohol, particularly if you are taking other medications.
- **Vision or hearing**. If you are not able to see or hear something clearly, it is harder to recall it. Have regular vision and hearing checks, and persist with wearing recommended glasses and/or hearing aids.
- **Anxiety and depression**.

I'm terrified of the future. What am I heading towards? I don't want to be a burden for my daughter.
Tom, 74, has dementia and lives with his daughter and her family

Like Tom, you may be anxious about becoming more dependent on others. It is helpful to focus on the present, and to do simple things that you enjoy—like walking or gardening—to help maintain a positive outlook and reduce your level of worry.

When I saw Terry, aged 68, he had just been diagnosed with Alzheimer's disease, after recently recovering from cancer treatment. He said, 'I have to concentrate on what I'm doing now. I don't worry about

5–10 years' time. I just do day-to-day stuff and I forget about what's going to happen in the future. I focus on the present. I enjoy spending time with my grandchildren.'

Anne

Feeling anxious about memory loss, and continually checking your-self for the next memory failure, can make memory loss worse.

If I think about my memory too much, it's worse. I have to be careful in conversation because I might say something that they don't under-stand. It worries me. I'm slipping and I know I am.

Isobel, 81, a retired secretary with dementia, does voluntary work at an opportunity shop

When you feel anxious, you might find it difficult to focus on incoming information. If you start feeling embarrassed, frustrated or worried about your memory, perhaps distract yourself by doing something else that gives you pleasure.

Sometimes you can't make your feelings of **anxiety** go away. Your fears and worrying thoughts might start to take over, and you might find it hard to relax. Anxiety can cause physical symp-toms, too—you might become more aware of your heart beating, feel tension or pain in your muscles, sweat more or breathe more quickly. If you notice these symptoms of anxiety for more than two weeks, it is important to seek medical assistance, as there are several effective treatments for anxiety.

I don't go to art group anymore because I feel vague, and I can't really put my mind to concentrating. I've lost my confidence and I'm not interested in the things I used to enjoy. I don't sleep very well and I'm often really tired. Why is this happening to me? What did I do to deserve this? My son is very worried about me, and it gets me down no end.

Carol, 74

Carol lives on her own and has early Alzheimer's disease. Her son describes her as having always been outgoing, bubbly and the centre of conversation, but now she is withdrawn. He says she always remembered friends' birthdays, but now forgets them, which upsets her. She has not been attending her usual activities. It is natural for Carol to feel sad, which is a common feeling when people have dementia. If you have persistent feelings of sadness for more than two weeks, you may have **depression**, so it is important to see your doctor. Common feelings when you have depression include feeling constantly down, useless or hopeless, irritable and moody, losing interest in life and being unable to enjoy things. When you are depressed you might have difficulty sleeping, eat too much or not enough, and have reduced energy. Symptoms of anxiety or depression are common when you have a memory illness like dementia. Your doctor may prescribe medication or refer you to see a psychiatrist or a psychologist for further assistance.

Lifestyle

As mentioned in Chapter 3, the way we live can affect our memory. Mental and social stimulation are important, but it's also important to get the balance right. If you are doing too much, and are **tired**, your memory can let you down more than usual.

Keep doing the things you enjoy, even if this means you have to modify them to take part. If you are still **working**, consider speaking to your employer about your illness and your symptoms. It may be possible to keep working, with some alterations to your work role. You might like to consider doing some voluntary work, or checking with your local council for regular social activities that you could take part in.

Joy was working as a stock-controller at a supermarket when she was diagnosed with Alzheimer's disease. She had done this job for nearly 25 years. Her friends at work had noticed that she was having memory lapses, and Joy was feeling anxious about her work performance. Her daughter suggested she talk to her boss about her illness and ask to do something else at the supermarket that did not require such keen memory, like stacking shelves.

Anne

I managed a bakery for 10 years, doing the paperwork, paying staff and working in the shop. I started to struggle with balancing the books and I felt constantly exhausted. I was asking the kids in the shop, 'Where's the butter?' or 'How long do we heat the pies for?' It was hard on the staff. I had to keep asking them all the time. They wrote out a chart with instructions, but it got too much, and I decided to leave. Now I'm helping with my husband's online retail business, packaging goods ready to be posted.

Mirka, 57, has Alzheimer's disease

Lorraine found that she could no longer play complex card games, such as solo and bridge, so her friends arranged for her to attend the local U3A (University of the Third Age) for regular lectures and social get-togethers.

Anne

I've played golf with my friends every Saturday for 30 years, but now I'm having trouble keeping track of my score, and my friends have to keep correcting my scoring. Last week I finally told them that I have Alzheimer's disease and they very kindly offered to do the scoring for me. Now I can relax and enjoy the game.

Rodney, 72

When you have a memory illness, you might find yourself withdrawing from social activities.

My social circle has slowly reduced.

Sarah, 72, has Alzheimer's disease

Sometimes people feel ashamed or worthless when they have dementia. Telling others your diagnosis may lead to a feeling of being stigmatised. Most people cannot understand what you are going through, so you can start to feel alone. If you do start to withdraw, you may feel even less confident about yourself because you start to lose your identity as a valued friend, group member or relative. It is important to maintain your social contacts and to share some of your concerns about the changes you are experiencing with trusted relatives or friends. It can provide a sense of relief to explain to others that there is a reason why you forget things. Dementia support organisations provide a range of opportunities to meet and talk with other people who have dementia. This can give you the chance to share with others who know how you feel.

I've 'outed' myself about my memory problem. It's good to have talked about it.
Ray, 83

Friends can react differently to the changes they see in you. However, some of your friends may find your problems something they don't want to know about, and withdraw.

I discovered, very painfully, early on that it is a mistake to tell friends.
Jim, 74

Jim found that some of his friends treated him differently after he told them about his dementia. They stopped asking for his opinion and no longer really listened to him, but Joan had a more positive experience.

Joan was always a very good tennis player, who played for a city club and a country club near her holiday home. She was diagnosed with Alzheimer's disease. Several members of her city tennis club became very frustrated with the changes they noticed in Joan's tennis abilities.

She forgot which side of the court she should be on and when it was her turn; however, her technical competence at hitting the ball and serving remained excellent. She was very hurt when officials suggested she no longer play. Fortunately, her friends at the country club were more tolerant. They found that if they reminded her when it was her turn, and which side she should stand on, she was still able to play well with them. She felt valued and respected by this group of women.
Anne

When you have dementia it can be difficult to keep track of conversations, especially when you are in a large group. Social activities that rely less on conversation and memory can be easier to take part in. These could involve attending a sport event, watching television, seeing a film or a show, going on a bushwalk or taking part in a group exercise session.

Handling frustration

The changes you are experiencing in your memory will affect you in a unique way. The type of memory illness that you have may be different from another person's, and cause varying symptoms. Many memory illnesses cause more difficulty with remembering recent events than things that happened in the past.

I can remember way back, but tell me something and ten seconds later I can't remember a thing.
Kevin, 88

When you have this type of memory problem, it is like your 'record button' for recording new memories is not working. It is not your fault: this part of your memory system has become less reliable and you are sometimes not able to 'record' new memories, even if the information is repeated and you try hard to remember it. You might forget what someone has told you, people's names, appointments, where you have put something, or have difficulty learning something new. This can be very frustrating and make you feel irritable, as it can pose a threat to your independence.

I do voluntary work at the local church. I feel bamboozled. I forget where I have put things, and must write things, like appointments, down on scraps of paper. I just can't keep it in—it just doesn't stay there. I'm not coping, I'm frustrated. My daughter helps, which is lucky. She helps a lot with my finances. I don't want to lose my memory; I want to boost it now.
Janet, 73

Using strategies for remembering

Using memory strategies means you can maintain as much independence as possible by lessening the load on your memory. This will help you feel more confident, and lessen some of the anxiety that often goes hand-in-hand with dementia.

Keep in mind that a memory illness doesn't necessarily cause difficulty in all areas of thinking. You will have **strengths** to draw on; for example, many people find they do well with reading, writing, longstanding memories and general knowledge, and well-learned skills, such as painting, singing, dancing or bowling. It helps to focus on these strengths, and keep doing more of what you can do well. Play to your strengths!

I play the piano to ease my frustration. I can still do that well, and remember so many pieces.
Lyn, 77

I go for a walk with my dog everyday—I'm okay when I'm with my dog.
Bob, 85

I might have dementia, but I'm not going to let it get me down—I'm going to enjoy life as it is now!
Toula, 74

I'm doing the best I can with what I've got.
Alex, 82

Memory strategies that involve using your strengths to get around any problem areas work well. For example, if reading and writing are a strength, then you can write a note to remind you of something that you might usually forget, like the details of an appointment. In this way, you are compensating for what is lost, rather than attempting to restore your memory back to how it was before the dementia began. This is like using a crutch to help you walk when you have an injured leg. A memory 'crutch' will help you feel more confident that you will remember important information.

Other approaches to enhancing memory can involve completing repeated memory stimulation exercises (see Chapter 5 for more information about memory stimulation), or the use of complex memory improvement techniques (see Chapter 6 for more information about these mnemonic strategies). When you have dementia, these approaches may put too much stress on your memory, possibly leaving you feeling less confident and more anxious about your memory. We talked before about your 'record button' becoming unreliable because of your memory illness. If your record button is no longer working, it may be best to work around this problem. Be proactive, and set up a back-up for incoming information, in case you forget it.

You will probably find that you are already using a 'memory back-up system', with a variety of common-sense techniques, like writing things down, because you have naturally adapted to the changes in your memory.

I was already handling this—now it just has a name. I'll keep doing what I've already been doing. I feel much better now that I've got my notebook.
Wendy, 69, has Alzheimer's disease

The strategies that *you* use will be different from those used by someone else with memory loss. We all have personal preferences in strategy use, and have different needs for using them. Some of us have always used a diary, others prefer a noticeboard. You are more likely to continue using memory strategies if you build on those that have worked for you in the past.

When I was at work I used to carry a little notebook with me in my pocket. I stopped doing that when I retired, but I might start carrying one again now.

Tony, 84, retired businessman, has mixed Alzheimer's and vascular dementia

Your own best strategies for remembering

Before making changes to the memory strategies that you use, think about the following:

- What specific situations do you need memory strategies for? For example, remembering appointments, to take medication.
- What types of memory strategies do you like using? For example, writing notes in a book, reminders in your mobile phone, getting your husband to remind you.
- Are you already using any memory strategies? For example, shopping list, calendar.

There will be various situations where memory strategies will help, so you will need not just one technique, but a whole range of strategies. You don't need to remember everything! Prioritise and work out what is important for *you* to remember.

Being organised with a regular weekly and daily routine can help reduce the load on your memory. There will be times when you need to rely on strategies more than other times—usually when you are dealing with any change to your lifestyle, like when you are on holidays, moving to a new house, or learning how to use a new piece of equipment. Be kind to yourself. Accept that some aspects of your memory and thinking have changed, and set realistic expectations. Allow extra time to do things that are new and complicated, and work on these tasks when you are feeling energised.

Your memory problem is likely to change with time, so you will need to make changes to the memory strategies you use, to adapt to any changes in the symptoms of your illness. When you have dementia, you have needs over and above those with milder memory inefficiencies so, while many of the memory strategies discussed in Chapter 6 are also relevant, it is worth elaborating on strategies that are particularly suitable for those with more significant memory issues. Chapter 9 describes ways that family members or carers can assist with strategies, and Chapter 10 outlines changes we can make as a community to support those with memory loss.

A memory centre in your home

Choose a special area of the house as your 'memory centre'. This area is your central point for storing information that needs to be remembered. Many people find the kitchen a good spot because it is somewhere they go regularly throughout the day and evening. You need to make it part of your everyday routine to regularly check your memory centre for reminders.

It works well to keep your phone in your memory centre, and have a notebook and pen ready to take notes while you are on the phone. Use a notebook rather than loose notes, as scraps of paper are easily lost! Keep your calendar or diary and a clock here, too. You could put up a whiteboard and/or pin board here. Keeping markers and pens attached to the board means you don't have to look for one when you need to write something down. Notes that are out of date need to be removed. It is best to keep the area simple and ordered, with no clutter. Perhaps someone else can help you set up and maintain this memory centre.

A memory centre can help you to remember:

- **Personal information**. You can have a section for permanent display, which could include names and phone numbers of people you see regularly (perhaps next to photographs of each person).
- **What day it is today.** Either you or someone else can write up today's date on the whiteboard, or mark off the days as they pass on a calendar. A clock or watch that shows the day and date is helpful. Another idea is to use a flip-top desk calendar and get into the routine of turning each day over and clipping it, when you come into the kitchen for breakfast. You can also check the day and date in the newspaper, or on your mobile phone or computer.
- **What time it is now**. Have your clock easily visible. A digital clock is often easier to read than a more traditional analogue clock.
- **Plans for the day or week**. Appointments, social activities, and things to do can be written on the whiteboard or calendar/diary, and crossed out when completed. This can also give you a record of your daily activities to look back on.
- **Things you need to buy or collect**. Update your list when you think of items you need. Remember to cross them off routinely as you put them away.
- **What to do in an emergency**. Keep a clear and separate list of emergency numbers by the phone. Include your address and a description of where you live, as it may be hard to recall these details under the stress of an emergency. Consider getting a push-button personal alarm system to wear around your neck, which is linked to a 24-hour emergency assistance service (it registers all your details automatically).
- **Phone numbers**. Attach a list of commonly used phone numbers near the phone, and regularly update the contact details for people stored in your phone. There are simplified phones available that can be programmed with a contact list display of regularly used phone numbers.
- **Phone messages**. If you use your phone near your memory centre, you can readily refer to your calendar, diary or notebook, and write messages straight into the appropriate places.

- **Medication**. Keep a list of your daily medication regime in your memory centre, too, as well as your medications, stored in an organised fashion. As suggested earlier, you could use a 'dosette box', a small plastic storage box for managing regular medications. The box is divided into compartments that allocate pills at particular intervals; for example, a weekly box with seven compartments, each holding one day's pills. Of course, the box has to be filled at weekly or other intervals, but it is simple to use and easy to check whether you have taken the necessary tablets. You may need to arrange for someone to help you load it up regularly. Alternatively, you could arrange for your pharmacist to make up a personalised foil blister pack ('Webster pack') of your medications once every week.

Marjorie, who lives at home by herself, was happy to get some advice about setting up a memory centre in her house. The first thing we did was clean up the clutter on her fridge door. She had fridge magnets from various tradespeople and emergency services from years back. We put the contacts that she used regularly in a prominent place, and got rid of the contacts that she no longer needed. We discovered she had both this year and last year's diaries on her phone table, and was often making entries in the wrong one. To avoid confusion, we put last year's diary away in a drawer, leaving only one diary accessible to write in.

Anne

You can carry a **smaller, portable memory centre** with you whenever you leave the house. A notebook works well, and could include the following information:

- identification details in case of emergency, including your name, address, phone number and emergency contact person
- a map showing where your home is, or the location of any other place you often visit
- important phone numbers.

Kevin has Alzheimer's disease. He retired from school teaching a year ago and now works part-time as a school caretaker, doing cleaning and painting. His wife gives him notes to take with him about the jobs he has to do each day, and he uses a diary with a pencil attached, which he always keeps in his top pocket. The diary helps him remember which days he is scheduled to work.

Anne

Writing things down

If I write things down, I don't feel so silly.

Owen, 74, has early Alzheimer's disease

Writing things down helps you to remember, as well as serving as a reminder. Keep as many of your reminder notes as possible in your memory centre. If you have notes stored in too many different places, you will have to remember where you put the notes! There will be times when reminders are needed away from the memory centre—so make sure that these written notes are easy to spot, accessible, and close to the to-be-remembered activity. For example, put a shopping list pad on the refrigerator or pantry door, or attach instructions for how to operate a piece of equipment on the equipment itself. Storage areas, such as cupboards and drawers, can be labelled with words or pictures that describe their contents.

I don't trust my memory. I have a small diary, which I take with me, and every day I need to check it. I also ask my family to remind me about things.

Alison, 69, has Alzheimer's disease, lives alone and does voluntary work

You can invite others to write reminders in your diary for you, and to make sure you write information down when they tell you some important details over the phone.

When I'm talking to someone and they say something that is important, and I want to remember it for later, I stop them and say, 'Hang on, I want to write that down so I can remember it later', and I get my notebook out and make a note straight away.

Stojan, 75

Finding things in their special place

Storing objects in specially designated places is helpful. Leaving objects in visible locations can act as a reminder to do something. Medications can be left somewhere obvious in the kitchen if they are to be taken with meals, such as on the kitchen bench. You can put medication next to your toothpaste if you have to take it in the morning and at night. A special place near the front door, such as a hall table, can be used to put things that you need to take out with you, such as a letter to be posted.

Work on dealing with the most commonly lost objects. For many people these items include:

- **Glasses/spectacles** can be worn around your neck on a glasses chain. Or you could have a brightly coloured box in each room for glasses storage, and make an effort to always leave your glasses in this box. If possible, have a spare pair of glasses as a back-up.
- **Wallets/handbags** can be stored in your memory centre, perhaps in a drawer or on a shelf nearest to your calendar, noticeboard, or where you keep your diary.
- **Keys** can be stored near the front door of your house. This makes it easy to pick up your keys when leaving the house, and to get into the habit of putting them back when you return. It can be helpful to make the keys more visible for easier finding, for example with a brightly coloured key ring. Keys themselves can be made of different colours, or have coloured 'covers' so particular keys can easily be picked out of a bunch. Have two or three sets of spare keys to leave with family members, friends or a

trusted neighbour. You might like to wear a frequently used key on a lanyard around your neck.

Location tracking devices can be stuck to frequently lost objects, enabling them to be found more easily. (See the section 'Alarms and technical devices' in Chapter 6 for details of tracking devices.)

Phillip, aged 86, has vascular dementia and lives in his daughter Julie's house. Julie is at work during the day, and when she gets home Phillip often can't remember where he has put his wallet or his keys. Julie decided to stick a location tracking device to her father's wallet and keys, so they don't have to have their daily search through the house!
Anne

Alarms and technical devices

Use **alarms** to remind you to do something. For example, set an oven timer to remind you to turn the oven off. You or a family member can program timed reminders into your smartphone, and type in details of what you want to be reminded of. For example, your phone can be programmed to sound an alert when you need to take your medication. You may want to ask someone else to help set up these more complicated reminder systems if you are not familiar with them. If you use a digital calendar on your smart-phone or computer, you can set this up to provide a variety of reminders, and share or 'synchronise' your calendar with others, so they are aware of your planned commitments. (See Chapter 6 for more information about technical devices.)

Consider using specially designed **'memory-wise' household equipment** to take the load off your memory. Many electrical appliances, such as irons and kettles, now have built-in shut-off devices in case the appliance is not switched off by the user. Safety cut-off switches can also be installed in gas stovetops, and special devices can be used to turn household lights on and off. Your local dementia support organisation will be able to offer further information about using assistive technology to support memory.

In Julie's kitchen she only has appliances that automatically turn themselves off after a period of time, in case Philip forgets to turn them off when she is at work.

Anne

Someone to help

Another way to take the load off your memory is to ask someone to remind you. Family members or friends can provide reminders for specific needs; for example, you could ask someone to call or text you to remind you of an important appointment, or to take your medication. Sometimes people arrange for nurses to visit the house to dispense their medication. Friends or family can also help with the upkeep of your home memory centre, making sure it is up to date, and writing up new reminders as required.

My family helps with my memory if they see I'm going wrong. If my wife goes out, she puts it on the board and I just look at it. I don't write notes myself, but I do write down phone messages.

Carl, 79

When family members write a note about where they are going, make sure they write down the day and date, exactly where they are going, the time they are leaving and the time they will return, and a phone number that you can call them on if you need to.

My memory fluctuates; some days I'm more alert than others. Some days I think, Why can't I cope? Oh, why didn't I remember that? I get annoyed with myself—I'm so silly, and I think my daughters would be disgusted with me about forgetting things. I write things down and use a calendar and diary too, but perhaps not as efficiently as I could. My grandson, Charlie, who is 18, is living with me at the moment. I often watch TV with him to distract myself from my worries.

Doris, 80

Doris would get more help from her written notes if she asked her grandson to remind her to use them. Using both a diary and a calendar can lead to problems, as you might not write your reminders on both. It works better if you have a streamlined system, with just one spot where you write your reminders. If you are out, and you don't have your paper diary with you but want to write a reminder, you can use the 'reminder' function on your mobile phone. Type in a message to yourself—one that will come up when you get home—telling you to make a note in your diary. Or if you don't use a mobile phone, ask someone to remind you to put the information into your home diary.

If you are going to an important appointment to discuss medical, financial or legal matters, it helps to take a family member or friend with you. If you do this, you can be sure that you provide all the information required at the appointment, and you will not forget any of the issues discussed, including the reasons why any important decisions were made.

There may be other occasions when you need assistance from others. You might be out for a walk and **suddenly feel lost**.

I can be somewhere and have no idea where I am. Everything that I am comfortable with is gone. I think, where the hell am I?
Roy, 66, has Alzheimer's disease

This feeling of disorientation is more likely to happen when you are somewhere unfamiliar, but it could also occur in familiar territory. If this happens, find someone to help you, and perhaps explain to them that you have a memory problem and need assistance. If you carry identification with you at all times, including your name, address, phone number and emergency contact, this will be helpful too. Some people like to wear a permanent bracelet engraved with their name, address, an emergency contact number and the words 'memory illness', in case of emergency. Another thing to consider is taking someone with you when you do go out, especially to some-where that you don't know well.

I keep my wife's phone number written on a piece of paper in my pocket when I go out for my daily walk.
Mario, 79, has Alzheimer's disease

A few times at the local shopping centre when I went to the toilet, I would come out and think, Oh God, how do I get back? I don't go to the toilets on my own anymore; I feel much more comfortable if someone comes with me.
Beatrice, 72, has Alzheimer's disease

Sally, aged 60, enjoyed regular lunches with her girlfriends for many years. She described a time when she suddenly felt lost:

This month's lunch was planned for a new location. I started driving there, but there was lots of traffic and I took several wrong turns. I just kept driving around and around and I got upset. I was running really late. I decided to pull the plug on the lunch and drove home again. It was a horrible feeling.
Sally, 60, has early Alzheimer's disease

Perhaps next time Sally has a lunch in an unfamiliar location, she could do some preparation before she leaves. She could draw a map, or write down her route so that she can check it as she drives, or pre-program the GPS in her car. Of course she could also ask a friend to accompany her or to pick her up.

When talking to people, it can be difficult to **find exactly the right word** to express what you want to say, which can make it hard to communicate. This is often worse if you are feeling anxious or distracted.

Nigel was having trouble recalling the name of the illness that his daughter had suffered from for most of her life. 'Oh, I know so well, but I can't say it . . . no I can't think of it . . . I know it so well.'
Anne

The word is there, but I can't access it.
Gina, 72, has Alzheimer's disease

Take your time—work on keeping calm, and if the word you are looking for still doesn't come to you, try:

- describing what you mean, using other words or gestures
- describing what it looks, feels or tastes like
- asking yourself, what do I use it for?
- showing someone what you mean by taking them to it or pointing to it
- drawing what you mean on a piece of paper
- changing the topic and coming back to it later
- getting rid of something distracting you, perhaps by moving to a different location.

Often it is helpful to be candid and tell the person you are talking to that you are having trouble finding a word; it takes the pressure off you, and perhaps the other person can guess. On the other hand, if that tends to fluster you, you might prefer to ask people politely but firmly not to prompt you, but to give you time to think—at least until you are ready to give up.

It may be helpful to talk to your family and close friends about how you like to handle the situation when you can't find the word that you want. Do you want them to say the word for you? Do you want to try and work it out for yourself, or use other words to describe what you mean? Of course, how you wish to manage a block for a certain word may change according to your energy levels and mood.

We all **value our independence**, and few of us like to rely on others for help. Karuni worked until she was 57 as a primary school teacher and teacher trainer, and now is a volunteer on her church committee.

It's my short-term memory; I forget things quite a lot, like what someone has just said to me. I can't recall a visit a few weeks ago. I have a pad on the dressing table and loose bits of paper. I've recently found I can't add up money, can't add up the little things. I've stopped driving. I think it's getting worse, and I hate to think I might get worse. It upsets me a lot. My older sister's memory is excellent; she is able to do everything. I'm reliant on her—she helps me to remember and she does the finances. I feel guilty asking for help, especially with something that I taught when I was a teacher.

Karuni, 72, has Alzheimer's disease

It is common to feel a sense of being 'nagged' when family and friends are providing regular reminders. Let people know when you can manage without their help, but accept the help you need. It often helps to tell people if the help they are giving you is too much at times. Ask them perhaps just to check what you have done, rather than to do it for you. You might like to find a place where you can have some personal quiet time, where you are not exposed to people's looks and reactions to your memory difficulties.

I've always had a great memory, and my husband has always had a bad memory. Now his is better and mine is worse. He is worried about me. He has taken over the shopping and finances and he wants to run the house like an army camp. We have a whiteboard and a shopping list book in the kitchen and a phone message book. He doesn't let me do anything by myself, and is always watching over me and being critical of what I do. I can do things like knitting, but I can't do it if something is distracting me, like when my husband puts the TV on really loud so

that he can hear it. He often tells me something when I am distracted and then gets angry when I don't remember it later. He is so impatient.
Amy, 76

I had difficulty just having quiet time in my shed because my wife always wanted to have me within her sight.
Fred, 79

It can be difficult to accept help from others, but this assistance often allows you to live more independently. Family members are usually pleased to be given the opportunity to 'give back' some of the support that you have given them over the years. It's often a case of 'what goes around comes around'!

Further information and support

Your family doctor can provide advice if you are concerned about memory. Your local dementia support organisation can provide further information, support and counselling. Details of such support organisations are provided in the 'Resources' section at the end of this book.

You might also like to check the services that your local council/health services provide. You can usually get help with cleaning and house maintenance, meals and transport. There is also a range of social activities or clubs to consider joining.

Key points   WHAT IF IT'S DEMENTIA?

- When people use the terms 'Alzheimer's disease' and 'dementia', they often use them interchangeably. Alzheimer's disease is by far the most common, but not the only, cause of dementia.

- Research into Alzheimer's disease continues to focus on prevention and treatment to slow or halt the decline, but so far no medical cure has been discovered.
- If the diagnosis is dementia, it helps to look closely at health and lifestyle issues and to use practical strategies to increase confidence, reduce anxiety, and work around the problems of memory loss.
- Useful memory strategies include: a memory centre in your home, writing things down, storing objects in special places, and making use of memory-wise household equipment.
- Asking someone to help with reminders and memory strategies is another way to take the load off your memory.

CHAPTER 9

Changes in someone else's memory—what can we do?

As our society becomes more alert to memory illnesses such as dementia, we begin to worry about other people's memory as well as our own. It can be difficult to know what to do if someone close to you is having memory problems. This chapter provides practical advice for supporting a family member or friend who is experiencing memory difficulties.

Normal age-related memory changes (Chapter 2) and health and lifestyle factors that can adversely influence memory from time to time (Chapter 3) have been discussed in previous chapters. It is possible that your relative or friend has memory inefficiencies related to being older, or to aspects of their current physical or mental health, or their living situation. For example, depression, anxiety, sleep deprivation, chronic pain or a major change, such as moving house, can all affect memory function. In addition, not paying attention to things is frequently related to not being able to remember them later. Some people may appear to be forgetting things, yet it may be due to their lack of interest or motivation to learn particular things. You might like to review Chapters 2 and 3 to check whether it seems wise to seek advice or treatment for any factors that you believe may be affecting your family member or friend's memory at the moment. You could suggest that your relative or friend reads this book, and together you could share ideas for everyday memory strategies, such as those suggested in Chapter 6. Talking about your strategies for remembering provides a good opportunity to think of new ways that any health and life-style factors can be better managed.

If you are concerned that there are signs of the beginnings of dementia, Chapter 8 provides information about dementia and Alzheimer's disease, including how memory loss related to dementia differs from normal memory difficulties, and how dementia is diagnosed. If the person you are concerned about talks to you openly about being forgetful, then suggesting a visit to the family doctor to discuss the memory issue is a useful first step. Referral to a specialist may then follow (see Chapter 8 for details of invest-igations typically completed by a memory specialist). Having a memory assessment and knowing what you are dealing with can really help.

For some people—and there are many reasons why—questioning or raising the issue of their memory abilities is not easy. Often people with memory loss are less aware of, and less concerned about, their memory than those around them. They might forget that they have forgotten something, which can be a difficult subject to broach. To further complicate matters, other family members or friends may have different opinions to you about the person you are concerned about. You will need to find a respectful, subtle approach that respects this person's dignity. Ideally, this will lead to discussing the problem directly, which will in the long run be a much more effective approach. Some people find it useful to make a time to see the family doctor on their own, to discuss the changes that they have observed in their relative. Others use a book like this one as a starting point for discussion. It can be a relief to finally talk openly about the memory problem.

It is frequently the case that adult children talk of their concerns about their mum or dad's memory with each other long before they raise the issue, upfront, with their parent. This is usually the stage when the family seeks professional advice.

Anne

Supporting someone who has memory difficulties

We are all different, and each person who has significant memory difficulties related to dementia or other changes in their brain is unique. When it comes to supporting someone with memory problems, there is no single correct approach, and the help that is relevant and effective can vary considerably. Often, there are changes in other areas of thinking and communication abilities, and in some aspects of behaviour and emotional control. The focus here is on memory, but it may help to talk with a doctor, health professional or counsellor from your local dementia support organisation about how to handle these additional changes.

Stop for a moment and think back to the last time you forgot something. You may have forgotten a particular word, what someone said to you, or where you had left something. How did you feel about forgetting this? How did people around you react to your forgetting? The way that we react to memory lapses is important.

Fergus, in his early sixties, came to see me to help work out what was causing his memory difficulties. He had only recently retired from a high-level management position. The consultation showed that Fergus had early-stage Alzheimer's disease with significant memory difficulties. As is often the case, Fergus was not fully aware of the extent of his memory issues and did not seem concerned about them. When I spoke to his wife, Carolyn, after completing my assessment, I was struck by her calm and caring manner. She was acutely aware of how significant her husband's memory loss was, and she knew it was likely he had the same illness that his mother and three of his mother's relatives had developed at a similar age. Carolyn gently described her husband's repetitive questioning and difficulty using household appliances that he had previously operated with ease. With a nurturing smile on her face, she put her hand on Fergus' arm and said, 'We just get through each day and don't worry about his memory problem.'

Anne

Fergus is fortunate to be living with someone who seems to understand that his memory difficulties are not his fault. They are related to a memory illness, and he doesn't forget things 'on purpose'. The way that we react to memory loss varies. If we can provide support in a calm and non-judgemental manner, then the person with memory difficulties is more likely to remain content. Of course, there are times when we lose our patience with a person close to us who has become repetitive or forgotten important things, which we know tends to amplify their irritability and anxiety about remembering.

Creating a supportive environment for someone with memory difficulties involves reducing the load on memory. It helps if you keep to a regular routine, doing things at regular times during the day and week as much as possible. Focus on familiarity—keep things where you have always kept them, shop at the same shops, and go for walks on well-known routes. Think about using technical devices that decrease the load on memory, such as appliances with automatic shut-off mechanisms, automated programs for timed sequences to switch lights on and off, and safety cut-off switches for kitchen appliances, such as gas stovetops.

When memory is a problem, many people feel challenged in social situations, and tend to avoid socialising. Your relative or friend will feel more comfortable with some people than others, depending on how people react to their memory difficulties. For them, keeping track in conversation can be a challenge, and talking in smaller groups or even just with one other person is often easier. At large noisy gatherings, arrange for different people to take turns spending time with the person in a quieter location, having a one-to-one conversation. Encourage your family member or friend to wear their glasses or hearing aids, if they use them. Avoid asking questions that rely on memory, such as, 'What did you do yesterday?' Instead, keep conversation in the here and now. If a person asks you the same question or tells you the same thing repeatedly, it may be best to try distracting them with another topic of conversation, rather than pointing out to them that they have already asked or said the same thing before.

You might need to talk more slowly and allow extra time for people with memory difficulties to respond. If they have difficulty finding the word that they want to say, you can help out by getting them to describe what they mean in other words, or asking them to show you or point to the thing they are talking about. If finding words is a regular problem, you might want to talk to each other about how it suits you both to handle this situation. Some people like to be told the word, whereas others like to try and think of the word themselves. People with memory difficulties can find it easier to socialise if they are doing things that don't involve as much conversation, such as watching sport, a film or a show, listening to singing or music, going for a walk or attending a group exercise session.

Play to the person's strengths

You might find that a relative or friend with memory difficulties talks a lot about things that happened in their past. These old memories are much stronger than memories of things that have happened recently (see Chapter 1 for more information about 'lifetime memories'). It's a good idea to make the most of these stronger memories, and help a person 'play to their strengths' to enhance their self-esteem and confidence. Encourage your family member or friend to keep up activities based on previous interests—these could be cooking, playing a musical instrument, gardening, playing golf, sewing, home maintenance, knitting, dancing, singing in a choir or painting. You may even want to ask them to teach you or others some of their well-learned skills.

Dad has pruned my roses with me every winter since I have had my own garden. He might have a few difficulties remembering where he has put things, and what people have said to him, but he is still an expert rose pruner! Each year I ask him to teach me more about pruning—it's a complicated process that he has learned over many years of experience.
Pam, 54

Mum was diagnosed with Alzheimer's disease a few months ago, but she can still play the piano. I've been tidying up our lounge room so that she can get to the piano easily. It brings us all so much joy when she plays, and she seems more relaxed when she is at the piano than she does at any other time.
Bruce, 51

I love watching Mum bake with my children, teaching them the same recipes that she taught me all those years ago. She radiates warmth and confidence, and delights in watching the kids tasting the goodies that they bake.
Mihiri, 55

Conversation with a person who has memory difficulties tends to flow more freely if the focus is on older memories. You can trigger reminiscence by putting on familiar music, or getting out some well-loved memorabilia or old photos. Some people like to research their family tree, or work on writing stories from their past that will be valued by generations to come.

For Dad's 70th we collected photos and had them made into a large album that we keep on the coffee table. There are photos from almost every year of his life. He loves it, and often looks through it with the grandchildren, telling them stories from when he was younger. For

Christmas I thought I would ask the older grandchildren to write down some of these stories, and we could add them to the photo album.
Eve, 49

Everyday memory strategies

We all use memory strategies in our own ways throughout our lives. When our memory becomes inefficient, we usually become more reliant on reminder systems to serve as a back-up for our memory and make us feel more confident that we will remember important information. These systems reduce the demand on memory. The aim of developing everyday memory strategies for a person with memory difficulties is to promote their continued independence.

It may be difficult to know how to talk about memory strategies with your friend or family member. It is important that they do not feel patronised, 'put down' or embarrassed. You could empower them by saying that they have already adapted positively to many aspects of their memory problem. You could draw attention to any reminder systems that the person is already using, and highlight how useful these strategies have been. You can also share the techniques that you find useful as a way of introducing new options for better memory management. Perhaps read through some of the suggestions for strategies in this book together to see if any ideas appeal to your relative or friend.

Deidre introduced systems to support her husband John's memory whilst at the same time showing that she values him. She has always used a notebook for reminders, and she encouraged John to use one too, saying that it is normal to use a notebook, because she has done so for most of her life. Each day she shows John her own 'to do' list, and asks him to write things into his notebook, like she does. She also fills out a dosette box for both her and John, so he doesn't feel that he is alone in needing a reminder system for his medication. She gently guides him at the same time as appreciating his strengths. She regularly praises him for having built their house on his own, and for being such a good listener. John feels valued for his strengths, and his weaknesses are normalised and minimised.

Anne

The approach you use will be strongly influenced by the nature of your existing relationship, and the demands on your family member or friend's memory. You need to find out the typical things that he or she tends to forget, and develop strategies which will suit those specific situations, and work for that person.

Mandula was often confused about which night she would go to each adult child's house for dinner. Her family didn't want to talk directly to her about this because they thought she would take offence. In the end Mandula's children worked out a good way to get around the problem. They devised a weekly routine, so that dinner at each particular house was on a particular day of the week: Tuesday night was Suzie's house, and Thursday night was Trevor's house. This lessened the demand on their mother's memory, and achieved the desired result in a subtle and respectful way.

Anne

We all have different preferences when it comes to reminder systems. Some people like to have appointments written on a digital or paper-based calendar, while others prefer that someone reminds them about the appointment the day before. When someone's memory is unreliable, assume that they will need a reminder, and develop a system that works for everyone.

I don't think Dad likes it when I remind him about things he forgets, like appointments and remembering to bring certain things with him. I've found that an indirect approach works well. I phone him and work the reminder into the conversation. I might say, 'I am looking forward to our lunch at twelve o'clock today', or, 'I want to check if I did ask you to bring . . .?' These tactful reminders have helped to safeguard the quality of our relationship.

Miki, 61

When I arrange something with Mum over the phone, I tell her to write it down on her calendar while I am talking to her. I say, 'Okay, Mum, go to your calendar now, find Thursday 12 October, and now write down family dinner for Callum's birthday at Rhonda's house at 7 p.m.' I have to get her to write it down while I am talking to her because she will forget to write it down after we have finished talking on the phone.

Rhonda, 57

Last week I didn't write down about seeing a film with my friends. I forgot to go and they called me to ask where I was. My friend asked me what she could do to help me remember for next time. I told her to remind me to write it in on my calendar and she said she will also call me the day before to remind me.

Eleanor, 69, has early Alzheimer's disease

I write things down, but I forget to look at them.

Jake, 76, has vascular dementia

Jake may have never used written reminders when he was younger. It can be hard to develop a new routine. He will probably need help with setting up and maintaining his reminder system, and encouragement to check his notes at regular intervals during the day. People are more likely to look at their reminder notes if the notes are put in a visible location, such as the kitchen bench. This spot can serve as the 'memory centre' in the house. (See Chapter 8 for information about setting up a memory centre.)

If you leave a **reminder note**, make sure that what you write is specific. For example, a note saying 'back in 5 minutes' does not provide enough information. Write today's day and date on the note, where you are going, and the time that you expect to be back. You could even add your phone number so you can be called easily if necessary.

On our recent holiday my wife, Ilsa, didn't want to come on an early morning tour, so I planned to go on my own. She knew about the tour, as we had discussed it the day before. I left at 5.30 a.m. and said goodbye to her, but she was half asleep. When I got back a few hours later, she was all upset, and said, 'I didn't know where you were.' Next time, I'll leave a note for her, saying where I am and when I'll be back.
Johan, 72

Setting up a '**communication book**' or a shared diary can be helpful, especially when people live on their own. The idea is to have information shared and updated by family and friends. This shared information system can be digital or paper-based, and enables a team-based approach to maintaining a reminder system.

Written reminders can be used for remembering a whole range of things. Some people like to have their cupboards labelled so they know what is in them; others like to have step-by-step instructions stuck on household appliances, such as the television remote control or a new microwave oven, so that they can be sure they will use the appliance correctly.

Remembering to take **medications** can be a challenge when a person has memory difficulties, and it may take time to develop a medication reminder system that works for your relative or friend. You could try a combination of the following ideas:

- Keep a list of your relative or friend's daily medication regime somewhere accessible. You could also keep an updated list on a digital shared communication app.
- Keep the medication organised and in a visible location. People often have their own personalised methods of organising their tablets that they have used for many years. Some like to leave tablets in their original boxes, others have little

jars or containers that they sort them into. Others prefer to use a purchased dosette box, or get the pharmacist to make up a personalised blister pack containing the tablets separated into labelled compartments for specific times of the day.

- Some people keep their tablets stored near something else as a reminder—for example, next to your toothpaste if you have to take it in the morning and at night, or on the kitchen bench if tablets are to be taken with meals.

- Most people with memory difficulties require additional reminders to ensure that they have taken their medication. Audio and visual reminders can be programmed into smart-phones, or you can phone your relative each day to remind them to take their tablets. Another option is to arrange for a nurse to visit each day to dispense the medication.

There are an increasing number of **technological devices** being created to assist people who have memory difficulties. While younger adults are usually familiar with new technology, many older adults who have not grown up with such devices can find them confronting. Be extra patient, and adopt a trial-and-error approach when introducing new technological aids to your relative or friend with memory problems.

My wife, Parveen, is 68 and has been diagnosed with early dementia. She has always been one to lose things, especially her keys, but now she loses them at least twice a day. As a birthday present, our well-meaning son gave her a location tracking device. He attached the device to her keys and programmed it to sound an alarm every time her keys were more than a certain distance from her wallet. He was upset when he found out that his mother had taken the device off her keys. Parveen said she removed it because she didn't like the noise it made. I noticed that she seemed embarrassed when the alarm sounded when we were in company, and she couldn't remember how to turn the noise off. I also think the alarm kept reminding her about her memory problem, and she didn't like that.

Saji, 71

My wife, Sylvia, and I have been using smartphones for several years, but we only use them for phone calls and texting. Our son said that we could set up a calendar reminder system for Sylvia to remember her medical appointments, but I decided to keep things familiar for her, and send her text messages as reminders instead. This involves more work on my part, but it means Sylvia doesn't have to try to learn a new system, which I think would be difficult for her now that her memory is giving her so much trouble.

Warwick, 76

The thing that bothers my mother the most about her memory at the moment is that she forgets what day it is. We came up with a simple solution for this. Whenever she wants to know the day, she quickly looks at her phone, and there it is for her, along with the date, month and time of day!

Wang, 58

When memory becomes a problem, many people wonder if memory exercises will help to build up the memory function again.

I have always done the family finances. Should I get him to start doing them now to stimulate his memory?

Leona, 78

Should we teach Dad how to do Sudoku puzzles?

William, 55

Our brains need stimulation and we can feel good when we challenge ourselves. When someone has memory problems related to a memory illness, such as dementia, it is important to get the balance right when it comes to learning new things. If your dad has always enjoyed Sudoku puzzles and he is not feeling overwhelmed by them, then they are to be encouraged. On the other hand, if trying to learn how to do these puzzles makes him feel anxious, then it would be better to find a different activity for providing stimulation. It is important to stay mentally stimulated, but we have to be careful not to put people off by making the activities too confronting or too difficult.

My husband, Viktor, is 71, and last month he was diagnosed with Alzheimer's disease. He only retired from his work as a lawyer a year ago. I think he forgets things because he's not paying attention, and I'm worried that he's not using his brain enough. In his job he used to keep his mind active all the time, and I think he needs to try harder to pay attention, and do some brain training to get his memory going again.
Iris, 69

Memory stimulation exercises and apps are readily available, and many people enjoy completing regular sessions of 'brain training' (Chapter 5 has more information about brain stimulation). When a person has memory loss related to changes in the brain from dementia, like Viktor, mental stimulation can involve more effort than it would have done prior to the dementia. Viktor may be more comfortable taking part in mentally stimulating activities that have already been part of his routine, such as attending a music concert, playing golf or spending time with his grandchildren. Activities that involve doing exercise and spending time with others give the added bonus of social and physical stimulation.

Extra support when life gets complicated

Memory problems often first become noticeable when people are trying to handle something that is unfamiliar, like arranging an overseas holiday or moving house. You might notice that your relative or friend with memory difficulties struggles with managing complex jobs, such as overseeing their financial affairs like they used to, and you need to provide assistance with these tasks, or take them on yourself.

Memory thrives on routine, but life is complex, and when you have a memory illness it can be difficult to manage situations that are out of your usual routine. Memory difficulties can be exaggerated when a person is physically unwell, or has physical discomfort or pain. Anxiety, distress and depression can lead to increased memory inefficiency (see Chapter 8 for more information about anxiety and depression), as can fatigue, excess alcohol and some medications. It is important to arrange a medical review if you think your relative has additional physical or mental health issues. Organising and attending a big family event, going on holiday, being admitted to hospital or even attending a medical appointment can all provide a challenge. The demand on memory becomes much heavier at these times, and you might notice that your relative seems more confused, and you need to provide more support than usual.

At various times of our lives we have to manage the often complex **medical system**. It is usually not just one medical appointment that we need to attend, but several, including blood tests and X-rays. When we get on this medical merry-go-round, it is often at a time when we are stressed or unwell. Add to that the complication of a memory illness, and you have a challenge on your hands! If you can go to the appointment with your family member or friend, then you will be able to provide the doctor with information that might otherwise be forgotten. It also helps if you:

- Write the appointment details down on your relative's calendar. Include the name of the health professional and their role.
- Call your family member the day before as a reminder.
- Together with your relative, prepare a list of questions that you want to ask the doctor, or issues that you want to discuss. Some very organised people like to assemble a 'medical history' folder in which they keep all medical reports and results.

- Ask the doctor to write down any instructions, or write notes yourself during the consultation.

A **hospital admission** requires extra support, especially an unplanned, emergency admission.

Last week I went to visit a relative in hospital a few days after her operation. She has early dementia and has been living with family for the past six months. She had a sudden health problem that required emergency surgery. She could not recall why she was in hospital, how she got there, how long she had been there, which hospital she was in or what day it was. She kept asking repeatedly about this information. She seemed unsettled and anxious about not knowing these details. She wanted to sit up, but she didn't know how to make the back of her bed move with the special hand-held controller. She wanted to watch TV, but again, she had no idea how to turn the TV on. She was clearly feeling uncomfortable about not being able to perform these relatively simple tasks independently.

In this case, a few simple changes allowed my relative to feel a greater sense of control. We brought in a clock with the day and date on it, and put this on her over-bed table where she could see it. We gave her a brightly coloured notebook with a pen attached to it with hat elastic, so that she wouldn't lose or drop the pen. In the notebook, we wrote down the name and address of the hospital, the date that she was admitted and the details of her operation. We added the name of her doctor and important contact phone numbers. We wrote down what the doctors had told her about what she was allowed to eat. We labelled the TV and bed controllers and put them where she could easily find them. We even put labels on the vases of flowers around the room, so she knew who had given them to her.

My relative wrote in her notebook each day—who had visited her, instructions from the nurses, and symptoms that she wanted to tell her doctor about. Her initial confusion settled and by the end of her week in hospital she was once again beating us all at the card games she loves so much!

Anne

When you spend time in a rehabilitation setting, you meet several health professionals. If you have a memory illness, it is difficult to remember who everyone is, and what their names are.

When Dad was staying at the rehabilitation centre, we asked each member of his treating team if we could take a photo of them to hang on the wall in his room. We stuck all the photos on a large piece of paper, and wrote each person's name and their role in the rehab team under each photo. It helped *us* to remember the information, too!

Jessica, 60

Looking after yourself

When you are supporting someone who has memory difficulties, you need to look after yourself, too. Share the load as much as you can, and work on developing a support team. Keep other family members and close friends informed—and don't be afraid to ask them to provide assistance. Many people want to help, but don't know how best to do this. Let people know what they can do to support you.

Stan's golf friends have been incredibly helpful. He was about to give up golf. He said he wasn't enjoying it anymore because he couldn't remember where he hit the ball and he had difficulty keeping track of his shots for scoring. Together, we spoke to his friends and let them know that he was having trouble with his memory. Not only are they now helping him with scoring, they have arranged a roster and he is now being driven to and from golf each week. This has made a huge difference for me. I know that Stan is enjoying himself when he is there, and I get to have some precious time to myself each week.

Lesley, 74

Remember that your relative or friend with memory difficulties can help out with many things, and they will feel valued if they can give something back to you.

When I met Bruno who has early dementia, and his wife, Denise, I was impressed by the way that they supported and valued each other. Denise had hip pain after a hip replacement and was due to have her other hip operated on soon. Bruno said, 'I do the lifting and she does the thinking.' Bruno assists Denise physically, and she supports Bruno with his memory.

Anne

Even though Mum's memory is a real problem now, she is still there for me, as she always has been. Whenever she is at our house, she does all my ironing, and she spends time with the kids so that I can get some other things done.

Bronwyn, 46

Build in some regular time for you. Even if it's just for five minutes, do something that you enjoy each day. Stay connected with the people who are important to you. Look after your health, eat well and exercise regularly. When you are supporting someone who has a memory illness, there is often a sense of grief and loss, as a part of that person has changed. You have had to adjust your expectations of that person, and take on a different role in your relationship with them. These changes can leave you feeling sad, lonely, stressed, anxious and depressed. At times you can feel guilty if you have lost your patience with your relative or friend who has memory difficulties. Make time to talk things over with a trusted friend or family member on a regular basis. Consider talking to a health professional, such as a psychologist, doctor or counsellor from a dementia support organisation. Many people appreciate attending a group where they can talk with others who are supporting someone with a memory illness. See the 'Resources' section at the end of this book for a list of helpful organisations. Remember that you need to nurture yourself to be able to nurture someone else.

I look forward to my morning walk around our retirement village with my friend Judy. We've always been there for each other, and I feel refreshed and ready to start the day when I walk back into our house after talking things through with Judy.

Merna, 82

I spent some time talking to Ken and his wife, Margot, who has Alzheimer's disease. They described the frustration, fatigue and grief that they had experienced related to Margot's dementia. At the same time, they conveyed a sense of continued joy in their relationship, and they said it has been important for them to remember that 'each day is a new day'.

Anne

Key points   CHANGES IN SOMEONE ELSE'S MEMORY

- If you are concerned about a relative or friend's memory, first check if age-related changes or health and lifestyle factors could be influencing their memory in an adverse way, and seek advice or treatment for these factors if you think it is necessary.
- If you are concerned about dementia, read Chapter 8. You may want to suggest a visit to their doctor and possible referral to a specialist.
- If your relative or friend has a memory illness such as dementia, provide a supportive living environment, emphasising routine and activities that draw on the person's continued strengths.
- Develop a range of memory strategies to promote confidence and independence.

- Provide extra support when there are changes to routine or additional physical or mental health issues.
- Look after yourself, and ask friends, family and health professionals to be part of your support team.

CHAPTER 10

Towards a memory-wise community

We live in a constantly changing society. There is an ever-increasing amount of information available to us. Life is busy; the pace is fast. There is more to do and see—and more to remember.

Our physical environment changes. New freeways and train lines are created, so we have to learn new routes to travel. New shopping centres are built, or old ones are modernised. The shop that you went to last week has moved, or the supermarket has rearranged its aisles.

We move from one work environment to another more often, meeting new staff and adapting to modified procedures. Many older people move from their homes into alternative accommodation facilities. All this moving means there is more to learn, in a never-ending process of making the unfamiliar familiar.

We are constantly having new technology thrust upon us. New computer systems and devices, regular updates to online banking software and apps, alterations to the way we connect to the internet and store information, smart TVs, and revamped access to music and media. The way we communicate with each other has changed, with fewer phone calls and more messaging via text and email. We have to remember passwords, PINs, email addresses and longer phone numbers.

There is now less service as we are progressively made to do things that used to be done for us. We shop, book tickets, and access government agencies for benefits and health rebates online. When we go to the airport, we check in our own luggage and print our own boarding passes on devices that seem to be different every time we do this. At some restaurants we order our food on touch screens rather than talking to someone. We are required to adapt to all sorts of new aids to help people with disabilities, and be aware of new names for community and health services, and the municipalities in which we live.

Multiple changes such as these place an unprecedented demand on memory capacity. At work and at home, we are constantly finding we need to keep 'up to date', but there never seems to be enough time. Continuing education is in high demand, and has become a major focus of many workplaces. Not so long ago, people were able to consider that by early adulthood they had attained most of what they needed to know about their field of expertise. These days, it seems that knowing everything is impossible.

More people are experiencing changes in their memory

The way that we live can make our memory processes less efficient, and at any age we can experience fluctuations in our memory. Forgetting some information is a normal, adaptive part of memory, but at times we feel that we are forgetting too much information.

It is hard to learn new things when we are bombarded with constant distractions: notifications flashing on our screens, the sounds of personalised ringtones, the pressing need to check our devices for fear of missing out on the latest information. Multi-tasking in an effort to get more done in less time, we are typically surrounded by the noise and sight of people around us in shared spaces.

We do a lot—maybe too much. We work long hours and often spend additional hours commuting to and from work. When we get home, we remain connected to work via our devices. Many of us feel overwhelmed, tired and stressed. It's hard to focus when you're worried about something, feeling rushed, or thinking about other things you have to do.

When we're overloaded it's easy to slip into unhealthy and ineffective habits, and maybe we don't take as good care of the workings of our memory—our brain—as we should do. We come home from work exhausted, perhaps drink too much alcohol, and don't eat or sleep well. We don't make time for regular exercise, or going to the doctor for routine health checks. We may experience other health issues that can impact negatively on memory, such as pain, depression and anxiety.

Some people develop specific anxiety about memory. They become anxious because of a memory lapse. Then, because they are so conscious of their remembering abilities, they notice every memory lapse that they make, no matter how small. They become more anxious, and often don't tell anyone about their fear. The increasing anxiety means they are more likely to 'forget', due to poor attention. They then notice more memory lapses and, in turn, become more anxious.

In addition to social changes making more demands on the memory abilities of all members of industrialised, technically driven societies, there is a demographic shift: the proportion of older people in our community is increasing. This means there are more people experiencing normal age-related memory inefficiencies, and more people who are living with significant memory difficulties related to memory illnesses, such as dementia.

Many of us work beyond middle age, and the increased demand on memory and frequent distractions inherent in the way we live can exacerbate any memory changes associated with getting older. In the same way, memory difficulties that are related to memory illnesses can be more pronounced when there is an extra load on memory, further impacting upon family members and friends who support people with significant memory loss.

Talk about memory!

With more people in our community experiencing real memory change, it's surprising that many people do not openly discuss memory. There is increasing media coverage of dementia-related memory loss, often focusing on the latest research for reducing the risk of developing dementia, or potential medical cures. From time to time we hear about people who have extraordinary memory powers, or who develop complex mnemonic techniques and compete in memory championships. Less sensational, although just as intriguing and important to our lives, are the workings of day-to-day memory—but these are rarely talked about.

A communal fear of memory loss seems to make it a taboo subject. Yet, if there was more discussion about the fluctuations that a lot of us experience in our remembering, then the fear and anxiety surrounding everyday memory fluctuations would lessen. People would realise that many of us experience memory inefficiencies, especially as we get older, and that the occasional memory lapse doesn't mean you are developing dementia. People would be reassured that they are not 'the only ones' to experience fluctuations in their memory, and by talking to others, they might pick up some new ways to manage mild memory changes.

Talking about dementia more openly in our community would help to reduce persisting stigma about memory illnesses. Recent media coverage of well-known individuals who have depression and anxiety has encouraged others to talk about their mental health issues. Putting dementia on the community discussion agenda, and sharing stories about living with significant memory illnesses, would promote more widespread understanding of what it is like to have dementia, and also get us thinking as a community about

how we can provide ongoing support for people with dementia—
as well as their family members and friends.

Be realistic about memory

We need to stop putting unnecessary expectations on ourselves in
terms of our remembering. Our memory processes will not always
be 100 per cent perfect, and there are many reasons why. The way
that we react to our memory lapses is crucial. We need to be kind
to ourselves. There will be times when our memory doesn't work so
well, and we need to use our best strategies to support remembering.

I know now that whenever I get stressed, I lose things, because I'm
rushing and I'm not able to focus on where I put things. This year I've
had a lot of work-related stress, so I decided to take action on my
memory. I have attached location tracking devices to the things I keep
losing, which has at least got rid of the added stress that my faulty
memory was giving me.

Anu, 57

As family members and friends, we need to be realistic about what
we expect from the memory abilities of those close to us. If Anu
was a relative of yours, you would probably know that she loses
things when she gets overloaded and stressed. You could easily
get annoyed with her when she is not able to find something—
again!—or, you could choose to be patient with her and downplay
her forgetfulness, knowing that there is a reason why she has not
been able to focus.

As a community, we need to be aware of the considerable individual variation that exists in memory ability. People we associate
with could experience intermittent lapses and fluctuations in
memory related to health and lifestyle factors, age-related inefficiencies, or significant memory loss related to memory illnesses.
We need to accept that there is change in memory abilities around

us and, ideally, generate a culture which makes allowances and provides support for this. While older adults in our community may experience minor changes in the speed with which they can encode and retrieve information, we continue to rely on their experience, intuitive problem-solving skill and wisdom. We need to support our elders in the workplace, many of whom provide invaluable leadership to our society.

Pay attention to paying attention

The distractions in our lives are endless. They come both from within us and from things happening around us. Many of our memory lapses are not actual 'memory' lapses but, rather, they are lapses in attention, resulting from distraction. The information didn't get into memory storage because we didn't pay enough attention to it in the first place.

We need to reduce the distractions that are interfering with our ability to remember. This is hard to do, given the way our community operates. We are less 'present' than perhaps we used to be because we spend so much time trying to multi-task. When we are with people, we are often looking at our phones or thinking about the next thing that we need to do, in the midst of our conversation. It is no wonder we forget things that people say to us.

The incessant distraction in our society has led some to the practice of mindfulness in an attempt to regain present-mindedness. Mindfulness training aims to reduce mind wandering and distraction, thus allowing us to fully engage in whatever we are doing. If we can learn to focus on the present, and pay attention to paying attention, then we may recover some of the encoding ability that gets lost to distraction.

If we can process information deeply, and make it meaningful to us, we will have a better chance of recalling that information later on. Creating the mind space to successfully absorb information can be challenging, but there is much to be gained from making a conscious choice to slow down, reduce distractions and pay attention.

Reduce the load on memory

Ideally, our society should be responsive and proactive in enabling us to learn how to adapt to the constantly new situations we find ourselves in. This supportive approach is especially important for middle-aged and older people who may otherwise be 'left behind'. Positive ageing has become a community issue in many societies, as shown through parliamentary inquiries, provision of access to learning for older people, and the development of special community facilities for retirees in sport, the arts and travel. Older people will enjoy better emotional wellbeing if they can develop and maintain social networks. Their ability to remain independent relies on good recall for rules, timetables and procedures; otherwise their participation in everyday life is restricted.

As a community we can lessen the demand on everyday remembering by making alterations to our environment. We can work on turning some of those technological advances that at times bewilder us into advances that benefit us. Most of us cannot keep all the information that we need in our lives 'in our heads'. What we need are better ways to access information when it is required. We need a 'memory-wise society'. We need changes in our homes, workplaces and community as a whole that will reduce the amount of information we need to keep 'in our heads'.

There are already many 'memory-wise' examples around us, but we can always do better! We can make better use of signs. Where? Almost everywhere! Inside buildings: shopping centres, large department stores, hospitals, large office blocks. Outside buildings: at schools, universities, accommodation facilities, holiday units, public transport centres, car parks. On nature walks and tourist routes: consistent use of symbols and signage for names of streets, speed limits, children's crossings; signs to tell you where the toilets and drinking water taps are, and to warn drivers of various features on the road (speed humps, winding road, etc.).

Signs can take many forms. They can be pictorial, or written. Pictorial or symbolic signs are very powerful and are usually culturally universal. Digital signage can be updated easily, letting drivers know about changed road conditions, or commuters know which train station will be next. Location maps, with 'You are here' clearly marked on them, are useful, and of course our technical devices can always assist us with locating where we are, and how to get to where we want to go next. Some shopping centres have their own apps to use for location maps. For people with visual impairment, there are apps that provide verbal directions, and many signs now include spoken versions.

We can design places to make them memory-wise. It is easy to get lost in new environments. If we use special design features, we can make this less likely. Making each part of a large place unique in some way will help you to remember your way around it. If it all looks the same, it's easy to get lost. Coloured lines on the floor can be used to direct you around places, such as hospitals. Way-finding in hospitals is crucial, as we are usually not familiar with the layout of hospitals, and arrive feeling stressed as we rush to visit our sick relative or friend or try to locate the department we need to go to. Car parks can include colour coding to tell you what level you're on, and perhaps pictures, as well as numbers. Remembering that you are on the level with kangaroos painted all over it may come to you more easily than remembering you are on the third level. Residential care facilities that often cater to people with significant memory difficulties related to dementia can also be made more memory-wise by the use of familiar furniture, colour cues, appropriate signage and lighting.

Design of household or work-related appliances can be altered to place less demand on memory. Instruction booklets are a must with any new devices. They should set out the steps clearly, and be able to be displayed where the user can refer to them again and again. Written and pictorial instructions can be combined to reinforce memory. Instructions that are permanently displayed on objects are invaluable.

Medication can be packaged in ways that reduce the load on memory. Some packets are arranged like a calendar, to help keep track of your daily intake, and you can ask your pharmacist to make up a personalised dispenser packet. New car designs are including more and more memory-wise features. There are lights and special alarms that come on to remind you that you need more air in a tyre, directions on the digital dashboard for how to get to where you are driving to, and sensors to remind you not to drive into the car behind you as you park!

For many of us, our smartphones are our most important memory aids, providing portable access to an infinite amount of information, literally at our fingertips; some describe their phones as an extension of their brain! We no longer need to remember phone numbers, as they are conveniently stored in our contacts list, along with other information if we choose, such as people's home addresses, and the names of their family members. We can take photos with our phone to help us remember things, like where our car is parked or the name of the wine we had at dinner last night. Our phone can help us find the word we are looking for, or remind us that we have a doctor's appointment tomorrow at three o'clock!

Create time for creating

Reducing the load on memory doesn't mean that everyone should sit back and stop using their memories. In fact, the result should be quite the opposite. If we can rely on memory back-up systems in our environment to take the load off recall of more mundane aspects of our lives, then we will be able to use our memory for other more creative or interesting pursuits.

If, for example, it takes less mental effort to find your car in a car park because you remember easily where it is with the help of the kangaroos, then it will be easier to use your memory for other things, like remembering as you drive out of the car park what the guest speaker talked about at the function you just attended!

A memory-wise community

We live together as a community, and we all experience difficulty with our memory at some point in our lives. When we are young, we might find it hard to learn information for an exam at school; in middle age, we might forget where we put something because we didn't pay attention while we were doing it. As we get older, it can take longer to put new information into memory, and retrieve it when we want it; and because of our increasing age, there is greater risk of our developing memory illnesses, such as dementia.

As a community we need to accept that our combined memory abilities are not fail-safe, especially given the busy, multi-tasking lives we lead, while dealing with continual change. We need to talk to each other about our memory problems, so we know that others experience similar situations and we can share information about what helps. We need to be kind to ourselves when our memory lets us down, and be kind to others in the way we react to their memory difficulties. As a community, we need to be more present-minded in order to maximise our memory, and work on ways to decrease the continual distraction that results from the way we conduct our lives. We need to design everyday objects and our built environment so that they reduce the load on our already over-loaded memory processes, to enhance our confidence and promote continued connectedness and independence as we age. We need to acknowledge the wisdom of our elders and be grateful for all that we learn from their combined life experience.

Together, as a community, we can nurture and support our collective memory abilities. Let's make being memory-wise part of our individual and community thinking and, in so doing, seek to enhance the dignity and self-respect of every citizen, young and old.

Acknowledgements

One way to be memory-wise is to learn from the experience of others. Over the years, I have been fortunate to be surrounded by supportive mentors who have provided continued opportunities for learning. *Memory-wise* enables me to share this collective learning. I am indebted to Annette Barlow at Allen & Unwin for publishing this book, and to Angela Handley and the editorial team for their assistance and attention to detail.

Delys Sargeant recognised the need for people to know more about memory, and encouraged me to share my knowledge with the community. While writing *Memory-wise*, I've had flashbacks to working with Delys many years ago in her office at VicHealth, hearing the passion in her voice, and seeing her beautiful flowing handwriting on her note pad. This book contains many of Delys's anecdotes and words, thus preserving her essence and wisdom, so she can provide a lasting legacy to us all.

Back in 1989, David Ames employed me as a graduate neuropsychologist in the first public hospital memory clinic in Victoria. Five years later, he suggested that Delys consult me about her memory, which led to the creation of the previous version of this book, *Remembering Well*. David is an international expert in the field of dementia, and I am very thankful for his ongoing encouragement and guidance. He has generously given his time and expertise to reviewing the information about dementia in *Memory-wise*.

Thank you to the colleagues I have worked with in my clinical practice. I have learned so much from working with you all in the Cognitive Dementia and Assessment Service at the Royal Melbourne Hospital, the geriatric psychiatry units at the Peter James Centre and the Albert Road Clinic, and my private practice. Thank you to all the people I have consulted with in my clinical work. The time I have spent with you and your family members has enriched my understanding of memory. Thank you for sharing your stories and the many creative ideas you have developed for supporting memory in everyday life.

Knowledge is passed on both ways when you teach, and I have learned a great deal through teaching. Thank you to the many students I have worked with in their clinical training. Thank you to the organisations that have invited me to provide regular education sessions to the community, including Council on the Ageing, and Dementia Australia, and thanks also to the people who have attended these sessions.

Christina Bryant gave me the opportunity to conduct research into memory during menopause, and I am deeply grateful to her and to Glynda Kinsella, Fiona Judd, Ben Ong, Bei Bei, Martha Hickey, Kerryn Pike, Liz Rand and Liz Mullaly for their mentorship and guidance. Thank you to the women who volunteered their time for the research and shared their experience of memory at midlife.

I am grateful for my supportive friends who motivate me by valuing my work. Thank you to the Symons family, and to Fel, David, Catherine, Dasha, Mum, Dad, Maddie, Will and Elsa. Finally, thank you to Mick for being there every step of the way.

Resources

Details for these organisations and apps were correct at the time of publication, but it may be best to check these details before contacting them.

Helpful organisations

Australia

Dementia Australia
Provides support, information and services for people with dementia, their family and friends, and health professionals
Phone 1800 100 500
www.dementia.org.au

Council on the Ageing
Advances the rights, interests and futures of older Australians
Phone 02 6154 9740
www.cota.org.au

Carers Australia
Provides information and support for carers
Phone 1800 242 636
www.carersaustralia.com.au

My Aged Care
Provides access to Australian Government-funded services
Phone 1800 200 422
www.myagedcare.gov.au

Australian Psychological Society
Provides information about common mental health issues and access
to contact details of psychologists by location and area of expertise
Phone 1800 333 497
www.psychology.org.au

APS Find a Psychologist service:
www.findapsychologist.org.au

Beyond Blue
Provides support and information about mental health issues, such
as anxiety and depression
Phone 1300 224 636
www.beyondblue.org.au

Lifeline
Provides 24-hour counselling for crisis support and suicide prevention
Phone 13 11 14
www.lifeline.org.au

Australasian Menopause Society
Provides information about menopause and access to contact details
of doctors who specialise in women's health at midlife
Phone 03 9428 8738
www.menopause.org.au

Jean Hailes for Women's Health
Provides information and access to clinicians and research in women's
health
Phone 1800 532 642
www.jeanhailes.org.au

New Zealand

Alzheimers New Zealand
Provides support, information and services for people with dementia, their family and friends, and health professionals
Phone 0800 004 001
www.alzheimers.org.nz

Age Concern New Zealand
Provides information and access to services to promote the rights and wellbeing of older people
Phone 04 801 9338
www.ageconcern.org.nz

Mental Health Foundation of New Zealand
Provides information and support for people who experience mental illness and their family and friends
Phone 09 623 4812
www.mentalhealth.org.nz

Australasian Menopause Society
Provides information about menopause and access to contact details of doctors who specialise in women's health at midlife
Phone 03 9428 8738
www.menopause.org.au

United Kingdom

Age UK
Provides information and support for older adults
Phone 0800 678 1602
www.ageuk.org.uk

Alzheimer's Society
Provides information about dementia and links to local support and research projects

Phone 0300 222 1122
www.alzheimers.org.uk

Women's Health Concern
Provides advice and information to women of all ages about their
gynaecological and sexual health, wellbeing and lifestyle concerns
Phone 01628 890199
www.womens-health-concern.org

North America

Alzheimer's Association
Provides information about dementia and links to local support and
research projects
Phone 1 800 272 3900
www.alz.org

National Institute on Aging
Supports and conducts research on ageing, and provides informa-
tion for the health and wellbeing of older people
Phone 1 800 222 2225
www.nia.nih.gov

Mental Health America
Promotes mental health and provides information and support for
people who experience mental illness
Phone 1 800 969 6642
www.mentalhealthamerica.net

Alzheimer Society Canada
Provides support, information and services for people with dementia,
their family and friends, and health professionals
Phone 1 800 616 8816
www.alzheimer.ca

The North American Menopause Society
Promoting women's health at midlife and beyond
Phone 440/442-7550
www.menopause.org

Canadian Menopause Society
Advancing the health of women at and beyond the menopause transition through education
Phone (604) 736-7267
www.sigmamenopause.com

Memory apps

The following links provide information about specific apps for supporting memory.

www.brainline.org/article/life-changing-apps-people-brain-injury

www.my-therappy.co.uk

https://otswithapps.com/ots-with-apps-mtool-kit-6-2-2013

www.tbistafftraining.info/SmartPhones/Phone_PHP/index.php

Notes

Chapter 1: How memory works

1   Ackerman, D. (1996). *A Natural History of the Senses*. London: Phoenix.
2   Anderson, M. (2015). Incidental forgetting. In A. Baddeley, M. Eysenck & M. Anderson. *Memory* (2nd edn, pp. 231–64). London; New York: Psychology Press, Taylor & Francis Group.

Chapter 2: How memory changes as we get older

1   Prince, M. et al. (2014). Dementia UK: Update Second Edition report produced by King's College London and the London School of Economics for the Alzheimer's Society www.dementiastatistics.org/stistics/prevalnce-by-age-in-the-uk/.
2   Toeppera, M. (2017). Dissociating normal aging from Alzheimer's disease: A view from cognitive neuroscience. *Journal of Alzheimer's Disease*, 57, 331–52.
3   Basak, C. & Zelinski, E.M. (2013). A hierarchical model of working memory and its change in healthy older adults. In T.P. Alloway & R.G. Alloway (eds), *Working Memory: The connected intelligence* (pp. 83–106). New York: Psychology Press.
4   Basak & Zelinski (2013). A hierarchical model of working memory and its change in healthy older adults. In *Working Memory* (pp. 83–106).
5   Verhaegen, C. & Poncelet, M. (2015). The effects of aging on the components of auditory–verbal short-term memory. *Psychologica Belgica*, 55(4), 175–95.
6   Drag, L.L. & Beiliauskas, L.A. (2010). Contemporary review 2009: Cognitive aging. *Journal of Geriatric Psychiatry & Neurology*, 23(2), 75–93.
7   Luo, L. & Craik, F.I.M. (2008). Aging and memory: A cognitive approach. *The Canadian Journal of Psychiatry*, 53(6), 346–53.

8   Luo & Craik (2008). Aging and memory. *The Canadian Journal of Psychiatry*, 53(6), 346–53.
9   Rose, S. (1993). No way to treat the mind. *New Scientist–UK Edition*, 138(1869), 23.
10   Meredith, A., Shafto, M.A., Burke, D.M., Stamatakis, E.A., Tam, P.P., Tyler, L.K. (2007). On the tip-of-the-tongue: Neural correlates of increased word-finding failures in normal aging. *Journal of Cognitive Neuroscience*, 19(12), 2060–70.
11   Nilsson, L. (2003). Memory function in normal aging. *Acta Neurolologica Scandinavica*, 107 (Suppl. 179), 7–12; Hedden, T. & Gabrieli, J.D.E. (2004). Insights into the ageing mind: A view from cognitive neuroscience, *Nature Reviews Neuroscience*, 5, 87–97.

Chapter 3: What else affects memory? Health, attitude, lifestyle

1   Gulpers, B., Ramakers, I., Hamel, R., Köhler, S., Voshaar, G.O. & Verhey, F. (2016). Anxiety as a predictor for cognitive decline and dementia: A systematic review and meta-analysis. *American Journal of Geriatric Psychiatry*, 24(10), 823–42.
2   Bouazzaoui, B., Follenfant, A., Ric, F., Fay, S., Croizet, J-C., Atzeni, T. & Taconnat, L. (2016). Ageing-related stereotypes in memory: When the beliefs come true. *Memory*, 24(5), 659–68.
3   'A Consensus on the Brain Training Industry from the Scientific Community', Max Planck Institute for Human Development and Stanford Center on Longevity, accessed 11 October 2018, http://longevity3.stanford.edu/blog/2014/10/15/the-consensus-on-the-brain-training-industry-from-the-scientific-community/; Lillard, A.S. & Erisir, A. (2011). Old dogs learning new tricks: Neuroplasticity beyond the juvenile period. *Developmental Review*, 31(2011), 207–39.
4   Sindi, S., Hagman, G., Håkansson, K., Kulmala, J., Nilsen, C., Kåreholt, I. et al. (2017). Midlife work-related stress increases dementia risk in later life: The CAIDE 30-year study. *The Journals of Gerontology Series B, Psychological Sciences and Social Sciences*, 72(6), 1044–53.
5   Mikkelsen, K., Stojanovska, L., Polenakovic, M., Bosevski, M. & Apostolopoulos, V. (2017). Exercise and mental health. *Maturitas*, 106, 48–56.
6   Le Berre, A-P., Fama, R. & Sullivan, E.V. (2017). Executive functions, memory, and social cognitive deficits and recovery in chronic alcoholism: A critical review to inform future research. *Alcoholism: Clinical and experimental research*, 41(8), 1432–43.
7   Unkenstein, A.E., Bryant, C.A., Judd, F.K., Ong, B. & Kinsella, G.J. (2016). Understanding women's experience of memory over the menopausal transition: Subjective and objective memory in pre-, peri- and postmenopausal women. *Menopause*, 23(12), 1319–29.
8   Walker, M.P. (2009). The role of sleep in cognition and emotion. *The Year in Cognitive Neuroscience 2009: Annals of the New York Academy of Sciences*, 1156, 168–97.

9   Waters, F. & Bucks, R.S. (2011). Neuropsychological effects of sleep loss: Implications for neuropsychologists. *Journal of the International Neuropsychological Society*, 17, 571–86.

10 Austin, M-P., Mitchell, P. & Goodwin, G.M. (2001). Cognitive deficits in depression: Possible implications for functional neuropathology. *British Journal of Psychiatry*, 178, 200–6; Porter, R.J., Gallagher, P., Thompson, J.M. & Young, A. (2003). Neurocognitive impairment in drug-free patients with major depressive disorder. *British Journal of Psychiatry*, 182(3), 214–20.

11 Rich, J.B., Svoboda, E. & Brown, G.G. (2006). Diazepam-induced prospective memory impairment and its relation to retrospective memory, attention, and arousal. *Human Psychopharmacology Clinical and Experimental*, 21, 101–8.

Chapter 4: Memory during menopause

1   Unkenstein, A.E., Bryant, C.A., Judd, F.K., Ong, B. & Kinsella, G.J. (2016). Understanding women's experience of memory over the menopausal transition: Subjective and objective memory in pre-, peri- and postmenopausal women. *Menopause*, 23(12), 1319–29.

2   Mitchell, E.S. & Woods, N.F. (2001). Midlife women's attributions about perceived memory changes: Observations from the Seattle Midlife Women's Health Study. *Journal of Women's Health and Gender Based Medicine*, 10, 351–62; Schaafsma, M., Homewood, J. & Taylor, A. (2010). Subjective cognitive complaints at menopause associated with declines in performance of verbal memory and attentional processes. *Climacteric*, 13, 84–98; Weber, M. & Mapstone, M. (2009). Memory complaints and memory performance in the menopausal transition. *Menopause*, 16, 694–700; Weber, M., Mapstone, M., Staskiewicz, J. & Maki, P.M. (2012). Reconciling subjective memory complaints with objective memory performance in the menopausal transition. *Menopause*, 19, 735–41.

3   van der Werf, S.P. & Vos, S.H. (2011). Memory worries and self-reported daily forgetfulness: A psychometric evaluation of the Dutch translation of the Multifactorial Memory Questionnaire. *The Clinical Neuropsychologist*, 25, 244–68.

4   van der Werf & Vos (2011). Memory worries and self-reported daily forgetfulness. *The Clinical Neuropsychologist*, 25, 244–68.

5   Gurvich, C., Hoy, K., Thomas, N. & Kulkarni, J. (2018). Sex differences and the influence of sex hormones on cognition through adulthood and the aging process. *Brain Sciences*, 8, 163; McEwen, B.S. (2014). Sex, stress and the brain: Interactive actions of hormones on the developing and adult brain. *Climacteric*, 17(Suppl. 2), 1–8.

6   Weber, M.T., Rubin, L.H. & Maki, P.M. (2013). Cognition in perimenopause: The effect of transition stage. *Menopause*, 20, 511–17; Epperson, C.N., Sammel, M.D. & Freeman, E.W. (2013). Menopause effects on verbal memory: Findings from a longitudinal community cohort. *Journal of Clinical Endocrinology and Metabolism*, 98, 3829–38.

7   Andreoletti, C., Veratti, B. & Lachman, M. (2006). Age differences in the relationship between anxiety and recall. *Aging & Mental Health*, 10(3), 265–71.
8   Griffiths, A., MacLennan, S.J. & Hassard, J. (2013). Menopause and work; An electronic survey of employees' attitudes in the UK. *Maturitas*, 76, 155–9.
9   Kinsella, G.J., Ames, D., Storey E., Ong, B., Pike, K.E., Saling, M.M. et al. (2016). Strategies for improving memory: A randomized trial of memory groups for older people, including those with mild cognitive impairment. *Journal of Alzheimer's Disease*, 49, 31–43.
10 Unkenstein, A., Bei, B. & Bryant, C. (2017). Enhancing memory self-efficacy during menopause through a group memory strategies program. *Menopause*, 24(5), 574–81.

Chapter 5: What can we do to reduce the risk of developing dementia?

1   Isaacson, R. (2017). Is Alzheimer's prevention possible today? *Journal of the American Geriatrics Society*, 65, 2153–4.
2   Livingston, G., Sommerlad, A., Orgeta, V., Costafreda, J.H., Huntley, J., Ames, D. et al. (2017). Dementia prevention, intervention and care. *Lancet*, 390(10113), 2673–734.
3   Isaacson, R. (2017). Is Alzheimer's prevention possible today? *Journal of the American Geriatrics Society*, 65, 2153–4.
4   Villemagne, V.L., Burnham, S., Bourgeat, P., Brown, B., Ellis, K.A., Salvado, O. et al. (2013). Amyloid β deposition, neurodegeneration and cognitive decline in sporadic Alzheimer's disease: A prospective cohort study. *Lancet Neurology*, 12, 357–67.
5   Isaacson, R. (2017). Is Alzheimer's prevention possible today? *Journal of the American Geriatrics Society*, 65, 2153–4.
6   Livingston, G. et al. (2017). Dementia prevention, intervention and care *Lancet*, 390(10113), 2673–734.
7   Livingston, G. et al. (2017). Dementia prevention, intervention and care. *Lancet*, 390(10113), 2673–734.
8   Galvin, J.E. (2017). Prevention of Alzheimer's disease: Lessons learned and applied. *Journal of the American Geriatrics Society*, 65, 2128–33.
9   Stern, Y. (2012). Cognitive reserve in ageing and Alzheimer's disease. *Lancet Neurology*, 11, 1006–12.
10 Lautenschlager, N.L., Cox, K., Hill, K.D., Pond, D., Ellis, K.A., Dow, B. et al. (2018). *Physical Activity Guidelines for Older Australians with Mild Cognitive Impairment or Subjective Cognitive Decline*. Melbourne: Dementia Collaborative Research Centres.
11 Livingston, G. et al. (2017). Dementia prevention, intervention, and care. *Lancet*, 390(10113), 2673–734.
12 Mikkelsen, K., Stojanovska, L., Polenakovic, M., Bosevski, M. & Apostolopoulos, V. (2017). Exercise and mental health, *Maturitas*, 106, 48–56.
13 Lautenschlager, N.L. et al. (2018). *Physical Activity Guidelines for Older Australians with Mild Cognitive Impairment or Subjective Cognitive Decline*.
14 Stern, Y. (2012). Cognitive reserve in ageing and Alzheimer's disease. *Lancet Neurology*, 11, 1006–12.

15 Lillard, A.S. & Erisir, A. (2011). Old dogs learning new tricks: Neuroplasticity beyond the juvenile period. *Developmental Review*, 31(2011), 207–39.

16 A Consensus on the Brain Training Industry from the Scientific Community, Max Planck Institute for Human Development and Stanford Center on Longevity, accessed 11 October 2018, http://longevity3.stanford.edu/blog/2014/10/15/the-consensus-on-the-brain-training-industry-from-the-scientific-community/; Owen, A.M., Hampshire, A., Grahn, J.A., Stenton, R., Dajani, S., Burns, A.S. et al. (2010). Putting brain training to the test. *Nature*, 465(7299), 775–8.

17 Livingston, G. et al. (2017). Dementia prevention, intervention and care. *Lancet*, 390(10113), 2673–734.

18 Livingston, G. et al. (2017). Dementia prevention, intervention and care. *Lancet*, 390(10113), 2673–734.

19 Dumas, J.A. (2017). Strategies for preventing cognitive decline in healthy older adults. *The Canadian Journal of Psychiatry*, 62(11), 754–60.

20 Gustafsona, D.R., Morrisc, M.C., Scarmeasd, N., Shahf, R.C. & Sijbeng, J. (2015). New perspectives on Alzheimer's disease and nutrition. *Journal of Alzheimer's Disease*, 46, 1111–27.

21 Livingston, G. et al. (2017). Dementia prevention, intervention and care. *Lancet*, 390(10113), 2673–734.

22 Walker, M.P. (2009). The role of sleep in cognition and emotion. *The Year in Cognitive Neuroscience 2009: Annals of the New York Academy of Sciences*, 1156, 168–97.

23 Waters, F. & Bucks, R.S. (2011). Neuropsychological effects of sleep loss: Implications for neuropsychologists. *Journal of the International Neuropsychological Society*, 17, 571–86.

24 Cross, N.E., Memarian, N., Duffy, S.L., Paquola, C., LaMonica, H., D'Rozario, A. et al. (2018). Structural brain correlates of obstructive sleep apnoea in older adults at risk for dementia. *European Respiratory Journal*, 52, 1800740.

Chapter 6: Strategies for everyday memory

1 Singer, G. & Singer L. (1994). *Making the Most of your Memory: Practical memory exercises for all ages*. Bundoora, Victoria: La Trobe University Press.

2 Bouazzaoui, B., Isingrini, M., Fay, S., Angel, L., Vanneste, S., Clarys, D. & Taconnat, L. (2010). Aging and self-reported internal and external memory strategy uses: The role of executive functioning. *Acta Psychologica*, 135, 59–66.

3 Kotler-Cope, S. & Camp, C.J. (1990). Memory interventions in aging populations. In E.A. Lovelace (ed.), *Aging and Cognition: Mental processes, self-awareness and interventions* (pp. 231–62). North Holland, Amsterdam & New York: Elsevier Science Publications.

4 Kinsella, G.J., Pike, K.E., Cavuoto, M.G. & Lee, S.D. (2018). Mild cognitive impairment and prospective memory: Translating the evidence into neuropsychological practice. *The Clinical Neuropsychologist*, 32(5), 960–80.

Chapter 8: What if it's dementia?

1   Bateman, R.J., Aisen, P.S., De Strooper, B.D., Fox, N.C., Lemere, C.A, Ringman, S.S. et al. (2011). Autosomal-dominant Alzheimer's disease: A review and proposal for the prevention of Alzheimer's disease. *Alzheimer's Research and Therapy*, 3(1).

2   Livingston, G., Sommerlad, A., Orgeta, V., Costafreda, J.H., Huntley, J., Ames, D. et al. (2017). Dementia prevention, intervention and care. *Lancet*, 390(10113), 2673–4.

3   Prince, M. et al. (2014). Dementia UK: Update Second Edition report produced by King's College London and the London School of Economics for the Alzheimer's Society, www.dementiastatistics.org/statistics/prevalence-by-age-in-the-uk/.

4   Gurvich, C., Hoy, K., Thomas, N. & Kulkarni, J. (2018). Sex differences and the influence of sex hormones on cognition through adulthood and the aging process. *Brain Sciences*, 8, 163.

5   Villemagne, V.L. et al. (2013). Amyloid β deposition, neurodegeneration and cognitive decline in sporadic Alzheimer's disease: A prospective cohort study. *Lancet Neurology*, 12, 357–67.

6   Gustafsona, D.R., Morrisc, M.C., Scarmeasd, N., Shahf, R.C. & Sijbeng, J. (2015). New perspectives on Alzheimer's disease and nutrition. *Journal of Alzheimer's Disease*, 46, 1111–27.

7   Cummings, J. (2017). Effect size of analysis of Souvenaid in patients with Alzheimer's disease. *Journal of Alzheimer's Disease*, 55(3), 1131–9; Soininen, H., Solomon, A., Visser, P.J., Hendrix, S.B., Blennow, K., Kivipelto, M. & Hartmann, T. (2017). 24-month intervention with a specific multinutrient in people with prodromal Alzheimer's disease (LipiDiDiet): A randomised, double-blind, controlled trial RSS. *Lancet Neurology*, 16(12), 965–75.

8   This figure was adapted from a figure in Kitwood, T. (1993). Person and process in dementia. *International Journal of Geriatric Psychiatry*, 8, 541–5.

Several of the quotations used in the text are drawn from Tripp, R.T. (1987). *The International Thesaurus of Quotations* (1st Perennial edn). New York: Perennial Library.

Index